WEIGHT LOSS

with

DIET
EXERCISE
STRESS REDUCTION

THE DES CONCEPTS TO ACHIEVE YOUR ULTIMATE HEALTH, WEIGHT LOSS, AND LIFESTYLE GOALS

NELSON A. BERRIOS, M.D.

DESCONCEPTS.COM

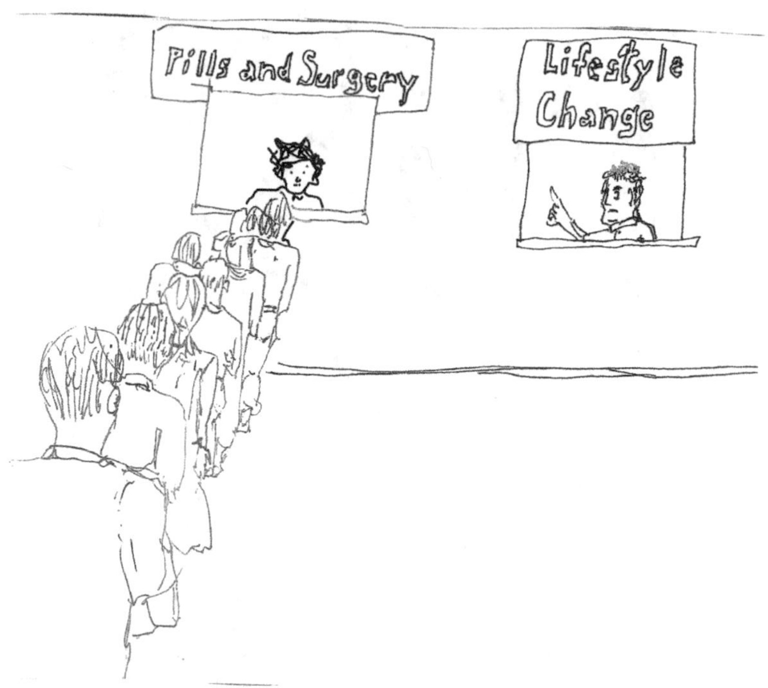

Pills and Surgery
Lifestyle Change

DESCONCEPTS.COM

TABLE OF CONTENTS

INTRODUCTION TO THE DES CONCEPTS 7

DIET..13

The Microbiome..14
BMI table 17
Inflammatory Foods:..20
Ultra-processed Foods 28
Mediterranean Diet..30
Diet by Age 37
The Glycemic Index 41
Resistant Starches 43
Timing of Meals, Exercise, and Fasting...........................45
Supplements 47

EXERCISE...65

Running 67
Walking 69
Resistance Training 73

STRESS REDUCTION 75

Spire TM...77
Meditation 78

DES CONCEPTS STEP ONE 83

DES CONCEPTS STEP TWO......................87

SLEEP..89

    Sleep apnea..90
    Circadian Rhythm.......................................93
    Sleep Hygiene...96

DES CONCEPTS STEP THREE 99

THE DES CONCEPTS BY
TARGET ORGANS 105

    Brain...106
    Gastrointestinal tract...............................113
    Musculoskeletal System..........................119
    Fibromyalgia..119
    Thyroid..121
    Type II Diabetes Mellitus.........................123

GLYCEMIC INDEX AND
GLYCEMIC LOAD TABLE......................127

SUMMARY OF THE
DES CONCEPTS................................135

APPENDIXES A – F 143

GLOSSARY 159

TIPS AND RECIPES 165

    Meatless Dishes.......................................190

DES CONCEPTS
REFERENCE SHEET 203

EXERCISE

*

DIABETES

HYPERTENSION

ELEVATED CHOLESTEROL

MEMORY LOSS, FATIGUE, DEPRESSION

WEIGHT GAIN, INSOMNIA, SLEEP APNEA, RESTLESS LEGS

GASTROINTESTINAL PROBLEMS, CONSTIPATION, DIARRHEA, MALABSORPSION

MUSCLE PAIN, FIBROMYALGIA, ATTENTION DEFICIT AND AUTISM SPECTRUM DISORDER

DIET

STRESS
REDUCTION

TRIANGLE OF HEALTH

Within the triangle we have a small sample of the illnesses we can control although not necessarily cure. There are certain modifiers that tend to work against our efforts. These include genetics, diseases, use of medications, and bad habits.

DES CONCEPTS

These letters stand for three pivotal aspects of health: diet, exercise, and stress reduction. As we explore these three aspects, we will have a clearer understanding of what it takes to maintain good health, longevity, weight control, and energy. Dietary control, exercise plans, and stress reduction help us look younger and live fuller more productive lives.

When discussing the aspects of diet, the first corner of the triangle of health, we deal with the balance of nutrients and the individual components of dietary intake including caloric and dietary needs. We will explore in more detail the various aspects of our Western diet. We will emphasize many of the negative characteristics of the Western diet and of course how to improve it. We will also discuss the poisons in our diet and how to make better food choices and maintain a better dietary balance. We will briefly discuss the concept of autoimmune diseases and how diet can affect these diseases. We will discuss supplements and how they can help or be of detriment to our health and discuss the role of the circadian rhythm in our quest for health which includes all of the components mentioned above. We will also discuss dietary differences between regions in different parts of the world.

The aspect that comprises the second corner of the triangle of health is exercise. Exercise seems to be more straightforward to most of us; do more of it, and you will reap the benefits. However, many times it is not as simple as it sounds. We need to discuss the type of exercise, duration of the exercise, what to do before and after and how to become involved in the exercise to remain motivated. Motivation is the hardest aspect to develop, and for exercise to work, it needs to be explored. How do we maintain motivation for something we do not necessarily enjoy? The answer is: you make exercise enjoyable! Find your passion; this seems to work for jobs and hobbies, so why not for exercise? You may like walking, swimming, and bicycling and you may have never considered running because it is too difficult. All these choices are yours and you can proceed to do it now as it is never too late to pick up an exercise program at any age.

Stress kills! And if it does not kill us, it will debilitate us, and destroy our psyche. We need to take control of our lives. There are some stressful aspects of our lives that we cannot change. More importantly, we need to find an outlet for this stress and not allow it to interfere with our well-being. We will discuss several aspects of stress reduction including meditation, yoga, and activities that can help reduce our daily stress.

We will also discuss sleep. Maybe the program should be called DESS, as sleep is primordial to good health. It appears that, if there are no disease processes related to sleep (such as sleep apnea), good sleep will occur naturally just by following the DES program.

 WEIGHT LOSS *with* DIET EXERCISE STRESS REDUCTION

Diets are difficult to follow, and many people will lose hundreds of pounds throughout their lifetime only to regain them. How do we deal with this dilemma? It is important to remember that if you don't know why you keep failing, you will continue to do so. You will see that I emphasize explaining the reason why we select certain foods over others. You will learn why different types of foods and vegetables are beneficial while others are not. You will learn that certain foods are detrimental to your health, which unfortunately is the basis of our Western diet.

Let us begin by describing the first 12 DES concepts. This will be followed by a description of the Western diet, the microbiome, obesity, artificial sweeteners, and genetically modified (GMO) products. Let us start with the first 12:

1. Diet changes can alter the microbiome.

2. Add prebiotics and probiotics to your diet.

3. Low carbohydrate diets outperform low-fat diets.

4. Eliminate all inflammatory foods.

5. Eliminate refined carbohydrates from the diet, or at least cut them to a minimum.

6. Sweeten only with monk fruit, Allulose or Stevia.

7. Eliminate all desserts.

8. Never drink a soda again, be it regular or diet.

9. Avoid GMO foods when possible.

10. Reducing the consumption of animal protein and fats can result in lower heart disease and stroke.

11. The best cooking oils based on all factors are avocado and olive oils.

12. Avoid excessive use of seed oils as they can promote inflammation.

Thus, we ask ourselves why do we have to make lifestyle changes? For many people, this is not even an issue as they exercise, get regular sleep, avoid high-stress situations, and eat healthily. But if I were to rank a percentage of the population who are actually in this group, I would have to sadly report that it is probably less than 20%. Approximately 42% of the US population is obese, and more than 9% have severe obesity. This has increased dramatically since 1999, when only 30% of the US population was obese and less than 5% were severely obese. It is now estimated that 51% of US adults will be obese by 2030. The prevalence of obesity is similar in both sexes. Still, it does seem to effect women more than men and does not discriminate against age as young, middle-aged, and older adults have similar obesity rates. There is some discrepancy as far as race as well. Non-Hispanic blacks have a rate of 50%, Hispanics have an obesity rate of 45 %, and non-Hispanic white people 42%. The non-Hispanic Asian people have a rate of only 17%. Obesity rates also increase with income and college education.

Changing to a healthy lifestyle lowers the risk of cognitive decline and of dementia. This also seems to counter any existing genetic risks a person may have. There are healthy lifestyle habits that could add more than a decade to a 50-year-old's life span. This would include maintaining a healthy weight, following a healthy diet, not smoking, regular physical activity and moderate alcohol intake. Following the Western diet and overworking can lead to early deaths. Studies have shown that more than 55 hours of work a week is associated with 33% increase in stroke and 13% increase in coronary artery disease. Our diets have changed significantly in the last few decades in a detrimental way and have resulted in a decrease in life expectancy. By following the DES concepts and adapting to the healthy lifestyle changes we can begin to undo some of the negative health effects.

By understanding the first 12 concepts you'll find some logic in the first step of the diet adjustment which we have called Step One.

Obesity is multifactorial and diet modification alone will not achieve the goals leading to a healthy lifestyle. That is why we have described this program as the DES concepts. Concepts guide diet, exercise, and stress reduction to make it easy to understand. We'll try to educate you on the rationale behind Step One and Step Two of the weight loss program. Step One is a cleansing diet, which is located on page 33. In order to proceed with the diet, you need to be ready physically and psychologically, convinced that the old ways of doing things are behind you. Step One is temporary. I recommend one week; however, I have had people stay on the diet for months at a time as they are inspired by the way the weight loss has occurred. Step Two, which is the DES lifetime diet, requires changes in habits, eating, exercise, and diet encompassing the multifactorial approach. This would include the exercise and stress reduction discussed in the latter section.

DIET

This aspect of the triangle is probably the most difficult to undertake and correct. Our Western diet has many negatives, among them:

- ➔ high caloric intake,
- ➔ high carbohydrate content,
- ➔ low nutritional value in processed and ultra-processed foods, and
- ➔ our tendency to overeat.

For example, dental disease is the most universal experience in modern man. An extensive survey held in 1919 revealed that European skulls from the Neolithic era were free from dental caries. What happened? The diet! To understand what happens in our bodies we must begin with the bacteria contained in our gut.

THE MICROBIOME (GUT-BRAIN CONNECTION)

Bacteria help digestion but, by the same token, may disrupt our bodily functions if we happen to have unfavorable (dysfunctional) gut bacteria. The microbiome is defined as a community of organisms that live together in any given habitat. This has long been discussed in medical literature, and, at first, was regarded as the bacterial flora and as the microbiota when discussing just the gut bacteria. The newer concept is that of the microbiome when discussed as part of the entire human body and its interactions. It has been shown that having the wrong bacterial flora can produce or enhance diseases. The gastrointestinal tract, where these bacteria, viruses, and yeast live, has long had a connection with the brain. We will sometimes refer to the gut as the second brain. This is the gut-brain connection. The best analogy that I can make is that of the worker ants and the Queen. The gut bacteria are the worker ants, and we can control them unlike the Queen. Many times, there is a revolt, and the workers take over. The best example is the donut on the plate. Our rational selves (the Queen) know that the donut is bad for you. However, some hidden powers (the gut bacteria?) entice us to eat the donut. Other factors go into this, including our addiction to sugar and unhealthy fats. When we indulge in one of these items, there are chemical signals sent to the reward centers of the brain (limbic system). The signals are part of a feedback loop that then provides reinforcement. We want to do this again! This is a survival mechanism that was needed before we created the supermarket so we could identify those foods that provided nourishment. It works so well (too well) with sugar; I could only wish we would get the same rush when eating a stalk of asparagus! The microbiome may also be involved in releasing chemicals, so the "Queen" will succumb to the will of the workers. The gut bacteria that reinforce this need to be changed.

1. Diet changes the microbiome.

2. Add probiotics and prebiotics to your diet.

When there is a dysfunctional microbiome, changes occur in the gastrointestinal tract that leads to inflammation, the breakdown of our immunity, and of the ability of the body to fight disease and repair itself. Factors that can destroy the harmony of the microbiome and lead to these changes include:

1. The use of antibiotics
2. Antibodies in livestock
3. Obesity
4. Stress
5. Pathogenic bacteria

Some factors maintain a healthy microbiota such as:

1. High fiber diet
2. Breast-feeding
3. Natural birth
4. Exposure to microbes
5. Consumption of probiotics
6. Favorable genetics

THE FOLLOWING IS A LIST OF PROBIOTICS AND PREBIOTIC FOODS:

PROBIOTIC FOODS

These are the good guys of the Microbiome and will help keep a healthy flora. They can increase the stimulation of the immune response, increase lactose tolerance and digestion, help intestinal microflora, decrease intestinal pH, decrease cholesterol, increase production of the B vitamins, decrease ammonia and certain toxins, and help heal the intestinal microflora after the use of antibiotics. They include:

- Kimchi
- Sauerkraut
- Yogurt
- Kefir
- Kombucha
- 70% chocolate(dark)
- Japanese Natto
- Some aged cheeses (gouda, cheddar, feta, provolone)

Prebiotic foods

Prebiotic foods are the ones that provide nourishment to the healthy microbiota. They include:

- Jicama
- Dandelion greens
- Garlic
- Chicory root
- Artichoke including Jerusalem artichoke
- Onions
- Radishes
- Leaks
- Asparagus
- Okra
- Carrots
- Mushrooms

Since we are rebuilding the microbiome, probiotics and prebiotics must be consumed on a regular basis. The excessive use of antibiotics, for instance, has been shown to increase the risk of breast cancer and diabetes. Excessive stress places undue pressure on the intestine and causes absorption problems leading to inflammation. The excessive use of proton pump inhibitors (the purple pill) has been known to increase hip fractures in the elderly, increase the incidence of pneumonia, and lead to B-12 deficiency. Acid suppression over months and years increases the risk of myocardial infarction (heart attack), increases the risk of hepatic (liver) cancers, and

   WEIGHT LOSS *with* DIET EXERCISE STRESS REDUCTION

dementia (Alzheimer's) and is associated with a shortened life expectancy. The microbiota plays an important role in controlling inflammation in the body and does this mainly in the regulation of the immune system by regulating the immune response. Approximately 70% of the immune system is located in the gastrointestinal tract, where most of our microbes live. Microbial cells outnumber human cells 99 to 1. Probiotics were found to suppress cytokine production (these are chemical mediators of inflammation) and intestinal inflammation. Specific probiotics, which are strains of live organisms, support a healthy intestine by reducing cytokine production. Dysbiosis (abnormal intestinal bacterial composition) and loss of diversity in the microbiota can be a sign of ill health or obesity. There is a bidirectional relationship between human microbiota and health. Dysbiosis can be correlated to inflammatory conditions that can affect a healthy immune system and promote inflammatory pathways.

OBESITY-BMI

Obesity itself is associated with gut inflammation and increased gut permeability. Obesity is also associated with hippocampal atrophy (memory banks of the brain), and this, in turn, with cognitive decline (memory loss). With chronic intestinal inflammation, we have a breakdown of the immune system as well as an increase in inflammatory chemicals not only in the gut itself, but elsewhere in the body, including the brain. This can result in a decrease in hippocampal neurogenesis (deficient brain cell regeneration) which increases the rate of mood disorders and dementia in people with chronic inflammatory bowel disease. Noxious factors can enhance the presence of inflammation in the gut with increased gut permeability (leaky gut), leading to inflammation in the brain. In addition, there is an increase in inflammatory factors in the gut with the concomitant use of nonsteroidal anti-inflammatory drugs (NSAIDs), ibuprofen, for example.

	LB	90	100	110	120	130	140	150	160	170	180	190	200	210	220	230	240	250	260	270	280	290
	KG	41	45	50	54	59	64	68	72	77	82	86	91	95	100	504	109	113	118	122	127	132
FT/IN	CM																					
4'8"	142.2	20	22	25	27	29	31	34	36	38	40	43	45	47	49	52	54	56	58	61	63	65
4'9"	144.7	19	22	24	26	28	30	32	35	37	39	41	43	45	48	50	52	54	56	58	61	63
4'10"	147.3	19	21	23	25	27	29	31	33	36	38	40	42	44	46	48	50	52	54	56	59	61
4'11"	149.8	18	20	22	24	26	28	30	32	34	36	38	40	42	44	46	48	51	53	55	57	59
5'0"	152.4	18	20	21	23	25	27	28	31	33	35	37	39	41	43	45	47	49	51	53	55	57
5'1"	154.9	17	19	21	23	25	26	28	30	32	34	36	38	40	42	43	45	47	49	51	53	55
5'2"	157.4	16	18	20	22	24	26	27	29	31	33	35	37	38	40	42	44	46	48	49	51	53
5'3"	160.0	16	18	19	21	23	25	27	28	30	32	34	35	37	39	41	43	44	46	48	50	51
5'4"	162.5	15	17	19	21	22	24	26	27	29	31	33	34	36	38	39	41	43	45	46	48	50
5'5"	165.1	15	17	18	20	22	23	25	27	28	30	32	33	35	37	38	40	42	43	45	47	48
5'6"	167.6	15	16	18	20	21	23	24	26	27	29	31	32	34	36	37	39	40	42	44	45	47
5'7"	170.1	14	16	17	19	20	22	24	25	27	28	30	31	33	34	35	38	39	41	42	44	45
5'8"	172.7	14	15	17	18	20	21	23	24	26	27	29	30	32	33	35	37	38	40	41	43	44
5'9"	175.2	13	15	16	17	19	21	22	24	25	27	28	30	31	33	34	35	37	38	40	41	43
5'10"	177.8	13	14	16	17	19	20	21	23	24	26	27	29	30	32	33	34	36	37	39	40	42
5'11"	180.3	13	14	15	17	18	20	21	22	24	25	27	28	29	31	32	33	35	36	38	39	40
6'0"	182.8	12	14	15	16	18	19	20	22	23	24	26	27	28	30	31	33	34	35	37	38	39
6'1"	185.4	12	13	15	16	17	18	20	21	22	24	25	26	28	21	30	32	33	34	21	37	38
6'2"	187.9	12	13	14	16	17	18	19	21	22	23	24	26	27	49	30	31	32	33	35	36	37
6'3"	190.5	11	13	14	15	16	18	19	20	21	23	24	25	45	48	29	30	31	33	34	35	36
6'4"	193.0	11	12	13	15	16	17	18	19	21	22	23	24	21	21	28	29	30	32	33	34	35
6'5"	195.5	21	12	13	14	15	17	18	19	20	21	23	24	47	49	27	28	30	31	31	33	34
6'6"	198.1	10	12	13	14	15	16	17	18	20	21	22	23	45	48	27	58	29	30	31	32	34
6'7"	200.6	10	11	12	14	15	16	17	18	19	20	21	23	21	21	26	27	28	29	30	32	33
6'8"	203.2	10	11	12	13	14	15	16	18	19	20	21	22	47	49	25	26	27	29	30	31	32
6'9"	205.7	10	11	12	13	14	15	16	17	18	19	20	21	45	48	25	26	27	28	29	30	31
6'10"	208.2	9	10	12	13	14	15	16	17	18	19	20	21	21	21	24	25	26	21	28	29	30
6'11"	210.8	9	10	11	12	13	14	15	16	17	18	19	20	21	22	23	25	26	27	28	29	30

Body mass index or BMI is a measure of relative weight based on an individual's mass and height.

Based on your BMI (height and weight), you can determine if you have a healthy weight. A BMI of less than 18.5 is classified as underweight. A BMI of 18.5 to 24.9 is considered a healthy weight. A BMI of 25 to 29.9 is considered overweight, and obesity is a BMI of 30 or higher. In our previous discussions of obesity, the definition was a BMI of 30 or higher. Low BMI has been associated with lower all-cause mortality. Higher BMI has been directly associated with heart failure risk, as has a lack of leisure time physical activity. High BMI has been associated with a higher risk for sleep disordered breathing (sleep apnea), acid reflux (heartburn), cancers, increased incidence of diabetes, hypertension, and more recently has been associated with memory decline.

However, obesity is a result of other processes that began years before. At one time in their lifetime, every obese person had a normal BMI. What happened? Let us go back to that time, or let us begin before the weight gain when we were in our 20s and 30s. Unfortunately, some people began even younger, as exemplified by the growing trend of adolescent obesity. Increased BMI through puberty and adolescence is associated with increased risk of adult stroke. The cause of this phenomenon is our diet. There may be a link between the presence of BPA found in many plastics and the onset of obesity. Some researchers think that artificial sweeteners may be at play and actually cause obesity. High caloric foods are readily available, and our lifestyle is so sedentary that weight gain is inevitable. There is somewhat of a scientific consensus that once you turn 40, your body composition and dynamics are such that you will begin to incur metabolic changes leading to disease. The tendency is to continue the unhealthy habits that eventually will lead to hypertension, pre-diabetes, and weight gain. I will call this phase " riding your genes to the end." You are trusting your genes to take you to your end- of- life.

3. Low carbohydrate diets outperform low-fat diets.

4. Eliminate all inflammatory foods.

There have been many diet fads that have come and gone, some emphasizing short-term changes that, for the most part, cannot be sustained. On the other hand, there have been other exceptionally good dietary guidance that suggests changing your entire way of eating that could be sustainable. Although there are several, they all have common ground. There is consensus on the limitation of carbohydrates (carbs) with an increase in vegetables and avoiding inflammatory foods.

PRO-INFLAMMATORY FOODS:

- Breads, rolls, baked goods
- Jams
- Candy
- Margarine
- Cake
- Molasses
- Cookies
- Muffins
- Cereals (except old-fashioned oatmeal)
- Noodles
- Cornstarch, cornbread
- Pancakes
- Corn syrup, corn cakes
- Pastry
- Crackers
- Pizza
- Croissants
- Popcorn
- Donuts
- Potatoes
- Eggrolls
- Potato chips
- Fast food
- Pudding
- French fries
- Relish
- Fruit juice
- Shortening
- Snack foods
- Soda
- Fried foods
- Sugar

→ Flour

→ Granola

→ Honey

→ Hotdogs

→ Pretzels

→ Ice cream

→ Tortillas

→ Waffles

Avoiding these foods will help heal the microbiome. High sugar and starchy food are high in calories and can make you gain weight. These foods can also make you look older.

Notice I did not mention fruit. I will come to this later. Unfortunately, radical diets encompass healthier food alternatives that are so difficult to follow, that most of us will not voluntarily try them unless there is a reward of some kind. For example: what makes the person with sleep apnea use a horrendous contraption covering his face and blowing air up his nose? The answer is the clearheaded feeling, alertness, and energy he gets the next morning upon awakening! Positive feedback will stimulate continued use. People who are overweight and have gastrointestinal problems, diabetes, hypertension, high cholesterol, arthritis, and other medical problems may find it easier to follow these radical diets as there is positive feedback with amelioration of symptoms and an overall feeling of well-being.

5.   Eliminate refined sugars from the diet.

6.   Sweeten with monk fruit, Allulose or Stevia.

7.   Eliminate all desserts.

8.   Never drink a soda again, be it regular or diet.

Thus far, we discussed how the use of antibiotics and certain medications can affect our gut bacteria. Other poisons in our diet interfere with the proper function of the microbiome. These would include:

→ Insecticides

→ Herbicides

→ Saturated fats

→ Trans fats

Artificial sweeteners (Splenda, NutraSweet, Sweet and Low, aspartame, sucralose, saccharin, etc.) can cause diabetes yet can be helpful for diabetics, can cause weight gain, yet can be used in weight loss programs. Other associations with the use of diet drinks include an increased incidence of stroke and Alzheimer's disease. Just one diet drink a day can increase that risk. So, who do we believe? Let us go back to the microbiome (gut bacteria). You just had a rewarding artificially sweetened drink that your dysfunctional microbiome wanted so badly. It tries to consume the sugars and, it cannot metabolize them because *it is not sugar it can use.* Your microbiome is now very angry and hungry. It dumps chemicals into the bloodstream to stimulate your appetite, and you overeat. The studies on weight gain on artificial sweeteners are very inconsistent. However, it was concluded that certain individuals do, in fact, gain weight when consuming diet drinks, and some do not. I can only guess that the ones with the dysfunctional microbiome are the ones that gain weight. Unfortunately, the studies were not geared toward this observation. Now let me be clear: *excessive use of sugar, artificial or natural, is associated with weight gain, diabetes, stroke, and heart disease. The use of artificial sweeteners is associated with increased risk of stroke and Alzheimer's disease.*

A dysfunctional microbiota can cause food toxins to enter the bloodstream, stimulate the immune system and spread inflammation. I would only advocate using monk fruit extract (without erythritol), Allulose, or Stevia, as these are natural sweeteners and not artificial. Recent studies have suggested that erythritol may contribute to heart disease.

Is the verdict still out as to the benefits of natural versus artificial sweeteners? So far, there has been no clear answer, but given the choices, using these natural sweeteners may be the better option.

9. Avoid GMO foods when possible.

GMO crops are a sensitive topic, with pundits debating either the benefits or detrimental effects of these products. On one end of the controversy, there is available evidence that indicates GMO foods are not harmful to humans. Genetic modification itself does not seem to make

GMO foods toxic or unsafe. On the other side of the argument there are claims that GMO foods are unstable. It is felt that, if anything, being able to spray your crops with glyphosate may be what causes harm to the human body. GMO crops can be sprayed with glyphosate (Roundup) to increase crop yield. Glyphosate seems to mimic certain hormones and can cause an increase in hormone-sensitive cancers. It also seems to deplete the body of some biologically active metals. It can interfere with the ability of the body to detoxify and get rid of certain toxins. As it is a potent antibiotic, it can cause damage to the microbiome, and it could also interfere with the synthesis of tryptophan and tyrosine, which are used by the gut for energy. Most of the canola, cotton, potatoes, soy, and corn in the United States have been genetically modified. If we eat processed foods, we are likely getting doses of genetically modified produce into our diets. Those against GMO products offer other claims including that altered genes remain in our bodies and are part of the microbiome. That means they are not eliminated, and affect not only the bacteria, but also our immune systems. They feel that altered genes can be transferred to the microbiome and, in turn, alter how we react to the changed microbiota. In addition to the effects of glyphosate, some genetically modified crops can be sprayed with toxins meant to keep insects away without affecting the plant itself; it was genetically modified to survive the toxin spray. Traces of those toxins have been found in humans.

It seems we are dealing with new concepts. Although genetic engineering may be part of the future of medicine and agriculture, there are so many unknowns at this time. I would strongly recommend avoiding GMO products if possible. Note that just like the toxins in the ocean, the little fish have little amounts of it; the big fish accumulate it as they eat more of the small fish. Likewise, poultry and beef that are fed GMO products will tend to accumulate it in their bodies. I have little doubt that there are people who can tolerate small amounts of GMO foods and glyphosate without any difficulty. But when it comes to disease, these chemicals may contribute to illness and should be avoided.

10. Reducing the consumption of animal protein and fats can result in lower heart disease and stroke.

11. The best cooking oils based on all factors are avocado and olive oils.

We need to reduce the amount of saturated fats and trans fats in our diets. There is clear evidence that saturated fats and trans fats increase cardiovascular events, heart attacks, and strokes. We should consume fats that are healthier for the human body, including cooking oils.

What are the healthiest cooking oils? First, it should be noted that oil (fat) carries more caloric density than most foods. What makes cooking oil healthy is the ratio of saturated fats to polyunsaturated fatty acids (PUFA) to the amount of monounsaturated fat (MUFA), the ratio of the oils. A good cooking oil needs to withstand high temperatures. Depending on the ratio, the oil could be solid or liquid. The ratio also can determine the effect on the human body. Exposing oils to heat and oxygen causes them to oxygenate and produce byproducts called " cooking oil polar compounds." These compounds may produce harmful effects on the body. Studies are now ongoing to determine if these risks are real. There have been studies that suggest overheating oil is detrimental to your health and can promote free radicals that, in turn, damage body cells by making changes in the DNA. When you use cooking oil at high temperatures even once, it can cause the breakdown of the double bonds in the oil and subsequent formation of harmful compounds. Furthermore, it has been suggested that cooking oils should not be reused and should be discarded after only one use. For cooking it is best to select oils with high MUFA ratios. Based on this ratio, the ranking of the cooking oils and the health factor is as follows: olive oil, flaxseed oil, canola oil, avocado oil, and walnut oil. These five seem to provide the best ratios. Of these, flaxseed oil provides more omega-3 and can be used in individuals with high blood pressure. Unfortunately, it becomes rancid very rapidly and must be stored in the fridge. The smoke point is relatively low at 225°F, so it should not be used for cooking. It can, however, be used for salads. Avocado oil has a high smoke point, and it is high in monounsaturated fats. It is also loaded with vitamin E. On the negative side, it tends to be expensive. Walnut oil, not unlike flaxseed oil, has a low smoke point and becomes rancid readily. It is high in omega-6 and Omega-3 in a favorable ratio.

Other oils that need mentioning include sesame seed oil, sunflower oil, and peanut oil. Sesame seed oil has a 50-50 ratio and a high smoke point but is low in nutrients. Peanut oil can sometimes be chemically extracted and be quite unhealthy. If you do use it, the label should say roasted, toasted, or expeller pressed. Sunflower oil has a high smoke point, but it is comprised mainly of omega-6 fatty acids, which are not as healthy. Corn oil also merits mentioning. It does have a high smoke point and may even help lower bad cholesterol levels. However, most corn grown in the United States is genetically modified (GMO), so the corn oil will be too. It also has a remarkably high omega-6 to omega-3 ratio of almost 50 to 1. A more favorable ratio should be 4 to 1. Other oils that may warrant mentioning and could potentially be harmful would include grape seed oil, soybean oil, and coconut oil. Grape seed oil can have harmful compounds in the oil due to the drying process, which involves direct contact with combustion gases. If you want to use grape seed oil buy organic. There have been some recent studies that suggest that certain substances in grape seeds may actually help promote longevity. Palm fruit oil may be healthy in other aspects, but it is high in saturated fat, which we need to avoid. Coconut oil is also high in saturated fats. Spray soybean oil is widely available. It is overrefined, and it is usually genetically modified (GMO). Based on all other factors, including if it is of GMO origin and smoke point, the two oils I recommend are olive and avocado oils.

12. Avoid seed oils as they can promote inflammation.

Unfortunately, nut and grain seeds are used to make oils, and these are high in omega-6, which can be healthy but, when consumed in high concentrations, can induce inflammation. The seeds used to make oil would include soybean, corn, canola, sunflower, safflower, and cottonseed oils. When consumed in excess, the omega-6 fats can increase inflammation and inflammatory disease. Note that omega-3 and omega-6 are essential fatty acids (essential because the body cannot manufacture them), so they must come from the diet. The omega-6 fatty acids are used primarily for energy (the most common is linoleic acid) and are important chemicals in the functioning of the immune system. It is the ratio of omega-6 to omega-3 that is important. The Western diet is rich in omega-6 oils in very high ratios 10:1 to 20:1 and higher. A more appropriate ratio would be 4:1 and even 2:1. Polyunsaturated fatty acids are unstable, and their oxidation releases free radicals. Free radicals cause inflammation. Chronic inflammation causes diabetes type II, heart disease, obesity, metabolic syndrome, irritable bowel syndrome, inflammatory bowel disease, macular degeneration, asthma, cancer, psychiatric disease, and autoimmune diseases.

High omega-6 foods also include chicken fat, pork fat, some nuts, margarine, commercial oils, and dressings. The reason the ratio is so high is that in order to obtain a significant amount of oil from the seeds you need a considerable number of seeds. This is not unlike fruit juices. In order to obtain an 8-ounce glass of juice you need to use large amounts of fruit. Although eating fruit and seeds is healthy, fruit juice without the fiber and seed oils without the rest of the seed is not. Nature never intended for us to **-eat two pounds of seeds-** in one sitting, which is what we do with just one tablespoon of seed oil. All fast food is made with seed oils, fried food is fried in seed oils, and salad dressings and sauces are made with seed oils. There is research that suggests that these seed oils seem to contribute to the onset of certain cancers.

We will soon begin discussing Step One of the DES cleanup diet. The cleansing of the microbiome will take some time and is somewhat difficult. However, once you understand the science and the rationale behind it, it is easier to follow.

   WEIGHT LOSS *with* DIET EXERCISE STRESS REDUCTION

THE NEXT 12 DES CONCEPTS ARE:

13. Eliminate ultra-processed foods.

14. The Mediterranean diet can be as useful as the DES lifetime diet, and it can be followed after the DES cleanup diet.

15. High-protein diets increase basic metabolic rate. This higher rate is temporary and will revert to normal as the protein load diminishes.

16. Start with the DES cleanup diet as it is easy to follow.

17. The DES cleanup diet is a modified Paleo diet.

18. Vegetarians live longer when they follow the DES principles.

19. A glass or two of red wine a day may offer invaluable benefits to your health.

20. The use of unsaturated fats, such as olive oil, can reduce the negative effects of the saturated fats in meat.

21. The use of red wine can help reduce the negative effects of saturated fats in the diet.

22. You need to change your eating habits as you age.

23. Adjust your diet as you enter a new stage in life.

24. High carbohydrate and calorie-dense diets are never acceptable at any age.

13. Eliminate ultra-processed foods.

Studies have found that consumption of ultra-processed foods is associated with an increased incidence of cancer and obesity. There are significant negative nutritional attributes of ultra-processed foods, which include high content of poor-quality fat, added sugar and salt, low vitamin density, and low fiber content. I have provided a list of ultra-processed foods.

ULTRA-PROCESSED FOODS

Four or more servings a day is associated with decreased life expectancy.

- Custard
- Flan
- Pudding
- Ice cream
- Ham
- Processed meat
- Chorizo
- Salami
- Mortadella
- Sausage
- Hamburger
- Morcilla
- Pate
- Foie-gras
- Meatballs
- Potato chips
- Breakfast cereals
- Pizza
- Pre-prepared pies
- Margarine
- Cookies
- Muffins
- Donuts
- Croissants
- Marzipan
- Carbonated drinks
- Artificially sweetened drinks
- Fruit drinks
- Distilled spirits (e.g., rum, gin, whiskey)

THE LEAKY GUT

As mentioned previously, the microbiota controls the overall health of the intestine including the tight junctions between the cells that line the gut. The term " leaky gut " is used to describe disruption of these tight junctions allowing abnormal proteins to enter the circulation. This, in turn, stimulates the immune system and causes inflammation. The bacteria and gut flora are responsible for maintaining these junctions and thus reducing the leak. They thrive on dietary fiber. With the DES lifelong diet, high-fiber carbohydrates and vegetables are introduced, the cornerstone to a healthy microbiome.

EATING HABITS OF CULTURES AROUND THE WORLD

It would be appropriate to begin this discussion by highlighting the five blue zones around the world. These are: Sardinia in Italy, Okinawa, Japan; Loma Linda, California; the isolated peninsula of Nicoya, Costa Rica; and the island of Ikaria, Greece. National Geographic Explorer and journalist Dan Buettner identified these areas. He used a blue pen to circle these areas on the world map. What is most important is to note that these areas are known for longevity. These individuals live well into the 90s and 100 years of age. They are genetically and culturally isolated. Their diet is plant-based and mainly consists of fish with occasional meat approximately 5 to 6 times a month. They consume dark, leafy greens, nuts, and olive oil. Grains will vary, but steel cut oatmeal, rice, and barley are all staples of these cultures. They do consume coffee up to 2 to 3 cups a day and whole grains.

14. The Mediterranean diet can be as useful as the DES lifetime diet. It can be followed after the DES cleanup diet.

Certain foods constitute the main staple food of certain cultures and countries. Corn is almost universal and can be consumed in different dishes and prepared in different ways depending on the culture. From Bourbon to corn on the cob, corn can be prepared in different ways,. It is used as masa, cornmeal, homini, grits and even a fermented version called sadza that is eaten in Zimbabwe. Rice can also be considered a universal food staple. It is consumed in the Caribbean, Asia, India, and the Americas. Similarly, wheat is also spread to be consumed universally. This is particularly true in Europe and the Americas. More regional food staples would include roots and tubers. Yams are consumed in West Africa, cassava in South America and West Africa, taro root in the Pacific islands, and potatoes are consumed in Europe and the Americas. Poi is consumed in Hawaii and consists of a thick paste made from taro boiled, mashed, and subsequently fermented. Starchy fruits are usually consumed in tropical countries and include plantain and breadfruit. Legumes are an especially important part of the diet in India, Africa, and Asia. In recent decades, the benefits of the Mediterranean diet have come to light. This diet is rich in vegetables, nuts, and whole grains and reduces the overall consumption of red meat. For most people, following this diet can reap health benefits by lowering blood pressure and cholesterol. It has been used in the treatment of memory loss, and with some modifications, in diabetic diets.

THE MEDITERRANEAN DIET

Although not as detailed and strict as the DES diet, the Mediterranean diet has been shown to improve diabetes, cholesterol, and slow the progression of Alzheimer's disease. People who follow the Mediterranean diet are less likely to have brain changes with the deposition of beta amyloid. Just like the DES diet, the Mediterranean diet has been shown to lower blood pressure, improve cholesterol levels and reduce inflammation throughout the body. Almost all the elements of the Mediterranean diet can be found in your local grocery stores. It emphasizes eating large amounts of vegetables, fruits and lean proteins and it is low in refined grains, added sugars and saturated fat.

   WEIGHT LOSS *with* DIET EXERCISE STRESS REDUCTION

WHAT TO EAT:

VEGETABLES. It should be the center of most meals and the more colorful the better.

FRUITS. Whole fruit (not fruit juices) for snacks and desserts and toppings for salads.

WHOLE GRAINS. Brown rice, 100% whole wheat pasta, and whole versions of other grains. If you are not gluten-sensitive, then whole grain wheat bread is an option.

OLIVE OIL. The main source of fat used for cooking and drizzling over dishes.

PLANT-BASED PROTEINS. This would include beans, soy protein, nuts, and legumes.

FISH OR OTHER SEAFOOD. It should be consumed 2 to 3 times a week.

WHAT TO AVOID:

SATURATED FATS. Beef is eaten only 3 to 4 times a month and is limited to 4 to 5 ounces.

REFINED GRAINS. White bread, white rice, and other processed grains.

ADDED SUGARS. This can be found in sodas, energy drinks, sweetened teas, sports drinks and other sweetened drinks. Also found in desserts.

STARTING THE CLEANSING OF THE MICROBIOME

Yes, the calories **in** have to equal the calories **out** for maintaining weight. Weight loss occurs when the calories out are more than the calories in. Weight gain occurs when calories in are more than the calories out. The problem is how do we do this. The human body is so resilient and adaptive that these in-and-out equations are useless.

Refined sugars have a very high glycemic index; they mimic pure glucose; thus, they raise blood sugars rapidly. These include granulated sugar, super-refined sugar as in sodas and sugary beverages, and powdered sugar. This also includes fruit juices. As mentioned previously, if you insist on using a sugar substitute, use only monk fruit, Allulose, or Stevia as these are derived from plants and not artificial.

15. High-protein diets increase basic metabolic rate. This higher rate is temporary and will revert to normal as the protein load diminishes.

For these reasons, I would start a diet based on salads and meat: the DES cleanup diet. It is easier for most people to follow, especially men. Since most are trying to control a chronic disease such as diabetes, brain fog, high cholesterol, migraines, fibromyalgia, arthritis, inflammatory bowel, acid reflux, memory loss, or fatigue, I will sometimes limit certain foods and add certain supplements. For now, we will stick to the basics and address individual illnesses later.

16. Start with the DES cleanup diet, as it makes it easier to follow.

17. The DES cleanup diet is a modified Paleo.

The cleanup diet can become boring after a while, and everyone eventually cheats. A slice of bread, a muffin, cake, cookies, pie, etc., and with this in mind, we need to modify the diet. We need to avoid inflammatory foods and ultra-processed foods. We also have to eliminate all desserts.

Now we are talking impossibility! The microbiome is at it again. Sugar addiction (yes addiction) is part of the problem. That is why starting the DES cleanup diet with no carbs will not starve you but will begin to clean up the carbohydrate mess you have in your gut. It makes it easier.

I really want to stay away from the supplement bandwagon, Still, if you have a difficult time dealing with this part of the diet, then you can use an amino acid used in the biosynthesis of proteins. The amino acid in question is L-glutamine and it is a non-essential amino acid, meaning the body can usually synthesize sufficient amounts of this amino acid. However, when the body is stressed (think microbiome and inflammation), the body's demand for it increases, and it must be obtained from diet or in this case as a supplement. Optional use of L-glutamine 500 mg to 2,000 mg daily may help with the sugar cravings.

We also need to take into consideration the fact that some people are used to high carbohydrate and high sugar meals. If you suddenly stop consuming high sugar foods, there may be an overreaction on the part of the body resulting in excess secretion of insulin and hence hypoglycemia (low blood sugar). As you start eliminating carbohydrates, which you will do abruptly, you may experience episodes of hypoglycemia. You need to be prepared for these by consuming small amounts of foods that could increase blood sugar quickly. If you are a diabetic, you need to monitor your blood sugars and adjust your hypoglycemic medications accordingly. This would include insulin and metformin.

You can avoid the potential of a hypoglycemic attack by having a sugar drink or food available and by adjusting your sugar lowering medications if you are diabetic. Metformin, as your lone hypoglycemic agent, does not appear to cause any problems.

A high quantity of vegetables and protein coupled with no or low carbohydrates seems very extreme. Vegetarians seem to miss part of the picture as they eliminate animal protein, but, let us be clear: they supposedly substitute with plant protein. Unfortunately, the part some of them miss is that they may consume a high carbohydrate load (high caloric content) and consume inflammatory foods. There is a false sense of security because they are not eating meat. They substitute carbohydrates for animal protein. They get sick when they reintroduce animal fat and protein into their diets. This is interpreted as being toxic to them when the flexible microbiome has changed, and they no longer have the microbiota to successfully digest animal fat and protein. A meat eater is given a high vegetable diet and they may have a difficult time finding the "palate pleasure" in it. It is the gut microbiome again. The palate pleasure of an avocado with broccoli sprouts drizzled in olive oil is very much enhanced in the vegetarian, who cannot figure out why meat eaters fail to appreciate the same pleasure. It is the microbiome. Diet can rapidly alter the human gut microbiome. Diets composed entirely of vegetable or animal products affect the gut microbiome altering its composition. Food borne microbes from both diets can colonize the gut and can include bacteria, fungi, and viruses. The gut microbiome can respond to the altered diet and contribute to the survival potential of the human race as an adaptive mechanism.

18. Vegetarians live longer when they follow DES principles.

19. A glass or two of red wine a day may offer invaluable benefits to your health.

This could get messy. This book is titled "The DES Concepts" and it is a lifestyle change. Diet is only one part of the triangle; exercise and stress reduction are the other two. Vegetarians, to their credit, are more dedicated to their beliefs and practice the DES concepts. However, they may not call it that. Vegetarians can reduce the risk of diabetes by 78% and the risk of hypertension by 75% compared to nonvegetarians. There is always an in-between diet where the consumption of meat (chicken, fish, dairy, and beef) is reduced. These semivegetarians can reduce the risk of diabetes by 28% and the risk of hypertension by 23%. Those who only eat

   WEIGHT LOSS *with* DIET EXERCISE STRESS REDUCTION

fish reduce the risk of diabetes by 51% and the risk of hypertension by 38%. When consuming only dairy, the risk of diabetes is reduced by 71% and the risk of hypertension by 55%!

So, it appears that meat eaters can do the same, but they need to follow the same DES concepts as vegetarians do and take precautions. There are antidotes for the saturated fat problem meat eaters face. Eating less meat is one of these options. This is one of the recommendations of the Mediterranean diet.

20. The use of unsaturated fats, such as olive oil, can reduce the negative effects of the saturated fats in meat.

A 2016 study in *JAMA of Internal Medicine*, demonstrated that after adjusting for major lifestyle and dietary risk factors, animal protein intake was not associated with increased mortality, but was associated with higher cardiovascular mortality. Plant protein was associated with lower all-cause mortality and decreased cardiovascular mortality. These associations were confined to participants with at least one unhealthy lifestyle factor which included smoking, alcohol intake, overweight or obesity, and physical inactivity. However, this was ***not*** evident among those without any of these risk factors. They concluded that high animal protein intake was associated with higher cardiovascular mortality. That high plant protein intake was inversely associated with cardiovascular mortality. That is why vegetarians have less atherosclerotic heart disease, which is the number one cause of death.

So, what is in meat that causes an increase in cardiovascular disease? It has been shown that depending on the specific dietary fat, certain foods can be associated with cardiovascular disease. This was noted in another 2016 article from *JAMA of Internal Medicine*. The findings in this article were that replacing saturated fat and trans-fats with unsaturated fats resulted in significant reduction of mortality rates from cardiovascular disease. Long-chain saturated fatty acids found in foods like steak, butter, and coconut oil, raise low-density lipoprotein levels, which is associated with cardiovascular disease.

You can reduce the cardiovascular risk imposed by saturated fats by drizzling olive oil on your steak. You can also reduce the total fat intake by trimming the meat before or after it is cooked, by using lean cuts of beef, and eating smaller portions.

RED WINE

21. The use of red wine can help reduce the negative effects of saturated fats in the diet.

There are many benefits to drinking red wine, and these can numerous. For instance, wine helps kill bad oral bacteria, may be good for circulation in the legs and keeps legs healthy. Compounds in grape seeds may combat Alzheimer's disease; a glass of wine a day may help with weight loss; it may help people with type II diabetes metabolize sugars and starches properly. Light and moderate drinkers have improved cognitive performance than nondrinkers; chemicals in red wine can cut the risk of the flu and may protect against influenza, especially after rigorous respiratory workouts. Wine can help heart health in later life and may keep women's bones strong. It may protect the brain cells from injury during stroke and other ailments such as Alzheimer's and Parkinson's disease. Resveratrol, a compound found naturally in red wine, seems to protect the prostate; low and steady doses of alcohol slowed the onset of rheumatoid arthritis in laboratory mice, may decrease the risk of heart attack in hypertensive men, may reduce the risk of lung cancer, and may increase longevity. There are numerous chemicals in red wine and some that we do not know about, that offer these benefits. Resveratrol is in the skin of the grape and needs to be in contact with the wine. That is why red wine has higher amounts of resveratrol than white wine. Interestingly, resveratrol is also present in dark chocolate. Another chemical in red wine includes quercetin which is a known anti-inflammatory found in the skins of fruits and vegetables. It is also present in apples and onions. Polyphenols, which are strong

   WEIGHT LOSS *with* DIET EXERCISE STRESS REDUCTION

antioxidants, also contribute to the anti-aging and longevity known to be associated with red wine drinking. The dilemma with drinking wine is usually the amount. I have seen definitions of mild, moderate, and severe alcohol consumption and these do vary depending on the expert. It is agreed that moderate drinking may consist of one to two glasses of wine a day. Some extended the definition to three glasses a day and some as far as three and a half. We agree that the amount of alcohol you can consume will depend on your size and how fast you metabolize the drinks. I feel that one to two glasses a day is enough and an occasional three will probably do very little harm.

DIET BY AGE

The next question is the inevitable "Will I ever eat carbs again?" The answer is yes, but not like you were eating them before. You see, your diet changes with practically every decade of your life. You eat differently when you are a baby than when you are 10 years of age.

22. You need to change your eating habits as you age.

A 70-year-old person eats differently than a 10-year-old. What is often missed is when these changes take place. Disease occurs when the transition is not made, for example, a 40-year-old eating like a 10-year-old. Now, he has hypertension, diabetes, high cholesterol, obesity, etc., to contend with, because he waited too long to make the dietary changes. The following figure simplifies this concept.

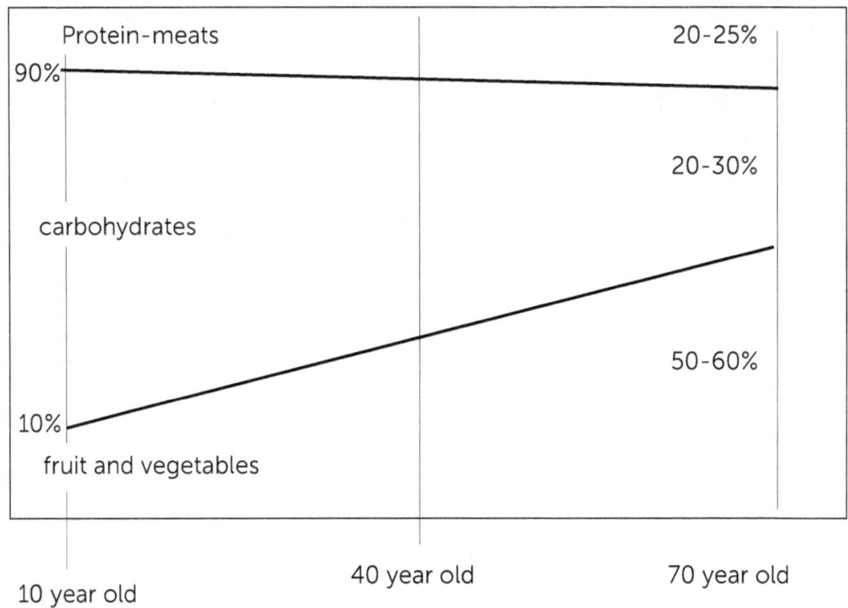

As much as I like the purity of the graph, it is still not correct. High caloric intake is needed when you are growing and procreating. These changes in diet occur in keeping with your stage of life as well as your age.

Calorie-dense food is an invention of modern society, and our microbiome and genetics have not adapted or changed fast enough to make these adjustments. Nature always finds a way if all those genomes that failed to adapt go on to succumb to these chronic illnesses, then the genetic pool will be rid of them. They will die off, the proverbial thinning of the herd. But alas! man has even found a way to cheat nature. Our advances in science and medicine now make it possible to keep everyone alive, even the sick ones. I even saw an article that stated they were working on a way to get all the benefits of exercising by taking a pill!

23. Adjust your diet as you enter a new stage in life.

24. High carbohydrate and calorie-dense diets are never acceptable at any age.

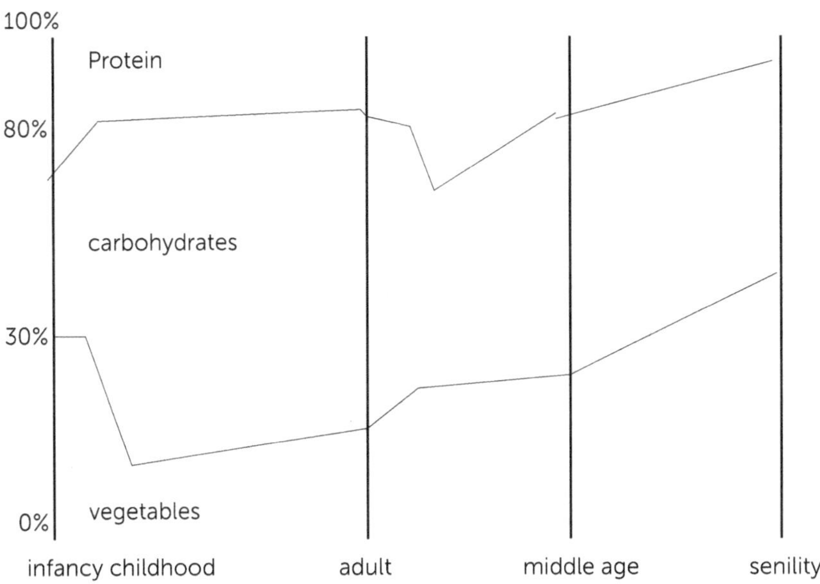

One of the first stages is the growing phase, after infancy. Then we procreate, then we enter middle age and finally senility, which for our purposes is after the age of 65. During each of these phases the amount of carbohydrates will vary. Protein consumption may increase during adult and mid-life but usually decreases in later life.

A recent article revealed that children may benefit from eating fish once or twice a week with an increase in IQ scores of almost 5 points. So, it is important to adjust all aspects of the diet not just the calories in or out, but the quality of the foods you eat. Eating sugary foods and carbs will destroy the palate of vegetables or fish as the microbiome is not cooperating.

The next 15 DES concepts are listed below. This will be followed by a discussion on the glycemic index, glycemic load, resistant starches, and genetics.

25. Introduce healthy carbohydrates slowly into the DES diet, preferably high in fiber and with a low glycemic index.

26. White sugar and high fructose corn syrup have an unacceptable glycemic index of over 70 and can lead to inflammation.

27. Genetics is only part of the picture. You need to follow healthy lifestyles (DES) to maximize longevity.

28. Consuming resistant starches will help with weight loss and fat burning.

29. Maximum benefits of exercise are best achieved when exercising in the mornings.

30. Partial and intermittent (16-24 hours) fasting may help in weight reduction, stimulate the formation of stem cells, help the immune system, and can be integrated into the DES.

31. If you want to eat breakfast, do so after exercise and make it the equal number of calories you just burned.

32. Reduce or eliminate gluten containing foods. Even if you do not have celiac disease, refined wheat is an inflammatory food and should be consumed in small amounts.

33. Taking supplements is optional; however, many factors alter and affect proper nutrition, and supplements can help offset these factors.

34. There are supplements that may help support a healthy microbiota, reduce anxiety and help sleep.

35. Some supplements may help with hot flashes, bone loss, and diabetes.

36. There is no single supplement that will cause weight loss.

37. Some supplements help joint pain, others can help stimulate your natural growth hormone levels, and some that may help improve memory.

38. Many supplements are detrimental to your health, especially when overdosing.

39. People with rheumatoid arthritis should be particularly careful with certain supplements which can actually cause more problems and worsen the disease.

GLYCEMIC INDEX

The glycemic index (GI) is a relative ranking of carbohydrates in foods according to how they affect blood glucose levels. Glucose is the pure sugar form and has a glycemic index of 100. We then compare other foods to this value. Carbohydrates with a low GI value of 55 or less, are more slowly digested and absorbed, thus causing a slower rise in blood sugar and insulin levels. Low GI carbohydrates are important for long-term health, reducing your risk for type II diabetes and of heart disease. It is also one of the keys to maintaining weight loss. It may even help control cholesterol levels when coupled with a high-fiber diet. For weight loss, a moderately high protein with low glycemic index diet is the best for long-term weight management. One way to find all-around healthy food choices is to look for the GI symbol. Unfortunately, it is not being used commonly. This symbol may be found in certain food products and can serve as a guide to finding low GI foods. Low GI foods are those that are less than 55, moderate is 55 to 69, and high GI are foods over 70. A list of the GI levels for some common foods is included at the end of the book. Sweeteners also have a GI. Those with a glycemic index of 70 or higher include white sugar, corn syrup, and high fructose corn syrup. Sweeteners with a GI of 65 to 54 include turbinado sugar (65), honey (60), blackstrap molasses (55), and maple syrup (54). Others worth mentioning would include barley malt, brown rice syrup, fructose, and agave syrup, all of which have GI levels less than 40. But note that they are still sugars, have a high glycemic load (>40), and need to be consumed in limited amounts.

25. Introduce healthy carbohydrates slowly into the DES diet, preferably high in fiber and with a low glycemic index.

26. White sugar and high fructose corn syrup have an unacceptable glycemic index of over 70 and can lead to inflammation.

GLYCEMIC LOAD

The glycemic load considers how much of the carbohydrate you are actually consuming per serving. Depending on the amount, it will have a proportional impact on the blood sugar level. Most diabetic diets are based on reducing the glycemic load. A low glycemic load is foods less than 10, moderate would be less than 19, and high glycemic loads are foods that are over 20. A list of GI and glycemic load for sample foods is located at the end of the book.

GENETICS

A man reaching 65 years of age today can expect to live until the age of 84-85. A woman turning 65 today can expect to live until age 86-87. Today, 25% of individuals over the age 65 will live past the age of 90 and one in 10 will live past 95. Some people live well into the 100s. There is a group of humans that live into the 12th decade known as super-centenarians. These individuals rarely face protracted illness or disability before dying. They have a genetic advantage it appears and it comes in part from having inherited less than the usual DNA variations known to raise the risk of heart disease, Alzheimer's, and other diseases. These individuals are uniformly healthier than centenarians in their final months and years. Rather than being lucky with the genetic codes, it is also possible that they possess DNA variations that actively protect them from aging. Attempting to decipher the genetic code of super-centenarians is an ongoing project by longevity researchers. Living to 90 or even 100 is too young when compared with the super-centenarians. If we are not lucky enough to inherit these genetic codes, then we must make the best of what we have. Even those who live to 110, cannot reach that goal on genetics alone. Genetics are the fertile ground in which diet, exercise, and stress reduction can cultivate longevity.

27. Genetics is only part of the picture. You need to follow healthy lifestyles (DES) to maximize longevity.

RESISTANT STARCHES

Resistant starches are not entirely digested, and travel through the digestive tract practically unchanged. The starch is resistant to digestion, hence the name. Starches are long chains of glucose that are found in root vegetables, grains, and different dietary foods. Resistant starches tend to help burn fat, make you feel fuller sooner, and decrease hunger. They also fill you up more as they are bulky food. They bypass the digestive system. They do not get absorbed. Cooking or heating destroys resistant starches, but you can recapture the resistant starch content of some foods by letting them cool after cooking. Butyrate (produced during fat burning) is thought to aid in protecting the gut from cancer, helping maintain a balanced pH, and help to boost the immune system. Some root vegetables are resistant starch foods (see Appendix A).

- Yams
- Jicama
- Pasta
- Sorghum
- Barley
- Persimmon
- Millet
- Celery Root
- Whole-Grain Bread
- Green Bananas and Plantains
- Navy Beans
- Pre-Cooked and **Cooled** Rice
- Oatmeal (Steel Cut)
- Taro Root
- Lentils
- Yucca
- Brown rice
- Tapioca
- Green Papaya
- Oats
- Farrow
- Quinoa
- Turnips
- Pre-Cooked and **Cooled** Potatoes
- Peas
- Pearl Barley
- Corn Tortillas
- Rice Pasta
- Cashews
- Mung Beans

28. Consuming resistant starches will help with weight loss and fat burning.

THE TIMING OF MEALS, EXERCISE, AND FASTING

You have followed the diet for a week, you are feeling much better, and you have lost nearly five pounds. As great as it sounds, it is simply inflammation along the gut and colon releasing fluids. The intestinal tract is 30 feet long, and the water retained during inflammation is slowly released as the inflammation in the gut subsides. Your microbiome has now changed. We need to recolonize it with new bacteria. In order to do this, you need to consume probiotics and prebiotics, out with the old and in with the new!

2. Add prebiotics and probiotics during the DES cleanup diet (this concept is worth repeating; see page 8).

When you reintroduce carbohydrates, they cannot be of the same type or amount you were consuming before you completed Step One of the diet. There will be a list of the favorable carbohydrates for you to choose with the Step Two diet.

29. Maximum benefits of exercise are best achieved when exercising in the mornings.

I recommend that exercise be performed in the mornings. Eat brunch after exercising. After the exercise you have burned your glycogen stores (stored sugar); if you wait another 60-90 minutes after the exercise before eating you will start to burn fat. You have fasted for about 16 to 17 hours which is an added benefit. There have been many benefits to the idea of fasting. Intermittent fasting encourages the natural repair systems to activate. It helps the immune system and stimulates stem cell proliferation. It should be noted, however, that fasting is not for everyone and in certain people it should be completely avoided. This would include pregnant women, breastfeeding mothers, people with a history of eating disorders, and, to a certain extent, the elderly.

30. Partial and intermittent (16-24 hours) fasting may help in weight reduction, stimulate the formation of stem cells, help the immune system, and can be integrated into the DES diet.

It seems that I have recommended skipping breakfast. If you want to eat breakfast do so after your exercise and make it equal to the number of calories you just burned, give or take. There has been a long-term controversy as breakfast has been represented as "the most important meal of the day." Studies have shown that eating breakfast results in higher caloric intake throughout the day and can result in weight gain.

I will add some controversy to the intermittent fasting theory. Proponents of the diet claim that intermittent fasting is a superior weight loss method. Researchers at UCSF and UHCC have found that some people who practice intermittent fasting experience a significant loss of lean muscle. The 2020 study stated, "Loss of lean mass and weight loss typically accounts for 20% to 30% of total weight loss. The proportion of lean mass loss in this study of approximately 65% far exceeds the normal range of 20% to 30%. The extent of lean mass lost during weight loss has been positively correlated with weight regain." The DES concepts do incorporate intermittent fasting, but the purpose is to burn fat, not to lose muscle. The body will use glucose, amino acids or protein, and fat as fuel. If you exercise at 80% or more of your exercise potential and you run out of your sugar stores, you will start burning protein and losing muscle mass to keep up the metabolic demand. The body will switch over to fat burning later. If you are performing intermittent fasting but are not utilizing energy sources at such a high level, and you have burned off your sugar reserves, you will burn fat first, but only for several hours.

31. If you want to eat breakfast, do so after exercise and make it the equal number of calories you just burned.

   WEIGHT LOSS *with* DIET EXERCISE STRESS REDUCTION

GLUTEN

We will be discussing gluten and its role in gastrointestinal disease later. But I would like to state a few facts about this protein. It is a group of proteins called prolamins and glutelins, which occur with starch in various cereal grains. Gluten is present in rye, barley, and wheat. Many times, other prolamins are also referred to as gluten, such as the hordeins in barley and secalins in rye. In people sensitive to gluten and those with Celiac disease, this protein needs to be eliminated from the diet.

32. Reduce or eliminate gluten-containing foods. Even if you do not have Celiac disease, wheat is an inflammatory food and should be consumed in small amounts.

SUPPLEMENTS

33. Taking supplements is optional; however, many factors alter and affect proper nutrition, and supplements can help offset these factors.

Humans have been on earth for approximately half a million years, yet supplements have been around for less than 80. Mankind has seen some people live into the 90s and 100s long before supplements were available. If you eat a balanced diet, you really do not need supplements. However, as well-balanced as our diets may be, we have already discussed that many habits, foods, and toxins interfere with proper maintenance of health. Is the absorption of certain nutrients being altered by a low-fiber diet? Do we have a dysfunctional microbiome? There are chemicals in our diets that may disrupt proper nutrient absorption, which we will discuss later. Are you blocking certain minerals with high phytate foods? Are the nightshades intoxicating the body? Is lectin causing absorption problems?

Many factors can alter and affect proper nutrition. Taking supplements is indeed a luxury, and to a certain degree, we should take advantage of this. Do you need to take a supplement for every bodily function? Of course not. The least we could do is consume probiotics and prebiotics on a regular basis to maintain a healthy microbiota. Certain supplements can assist in this goal. On the flip side of this argument is that many supplements may be contaminated with unknown and unwanted chemicals. The manufacturing of many supplements is unregulated, and they may not even be effective. It should also be noted that supplements may interfere with your other prescription medications. It goes without saying that the cost of these supplements can add up quite rapidly. Select a health topic that most interests you. If you have problems with diabetes because it runs in the family, it will help to use the supplements that help with diabetes. The same goes for supplements to help memory, weight loss, reduce stress and improve sleep. Our biggest concern at this juncture is that of gut and gastrointestinal inflammation.

34. There are supplements that help support a healthy microbiota, reduce anxiety, and help sleep.

FOR GUT HEALTH

The four main supplements for gut health, aside from the prebiotics and probiotics, would be **L-glutamine, berberine, curcumin, and L-tryptophan.**

Berberine is an herb found in Europe and Asia. It can lower cholesterol, lower blood sugar levels, modulate the gut microbiota, and prevent obesity. It can be added to probiotics, **magnesium** supplements, **DHA**, and **inulin** (that will act as a prebiotic). DHA (docosahexaenoic acid) is an omega-3 fatty acid that is the primary structural component of the brain, skin, and retina. It can be synthesized from alpha-lipoic acid (**ALA**), maternal milk, fish oil, or algae oil.

In addition to the above supplements, **curcumin** can help reduce gut inflammation. It would be quite beneficial in the early stages of DES cleanup. **L-tryptophan** supports gastrointestinal health and can also be taken at any time.

TO REDUCE STRESS

To reduce stress and depression, **selenium** and **magnesium** supplements may be helpful. **Passionflower** can reduce anxiety through certain chemical receptors in the brain. It contains chrysin, which is a strong antioxidant. Other stress-reducing supplements can be used to help sleep, as discussed below.

FOR SLEEP

Melatonin can be added to aid in poor sleep. I would start with 3 mg as it can be easily reduced by half or increased to 6 mg in order to find the correct dosage. Overdose of melatonin can produce daytime sleepiness, especially in the elderly. It does seem to increase dreaming to a certain degree. It has also been helpful for migraine prevention. Keep in mind that poor sleep is the result of an overstimulated brain, and insomnia is usually seen in anxious individuals. Any of the supplements that aid anxiety and stress will likewise aid in treating insomnia. Stress-reducing techniques will also be helpful. **Ashwagandha** reduces anxiety and contains withanolides, which is a steroidal lactone and acts through the GABA p1(rho) receptor. GABA is one of the neurotransmitters the body uses to turn off brain and nerve activity. **Chamomile** also contains flavonoids that help reduce anxiety and aid sleep. We can also add **magnolia** (tree bark) and **green tea** to the list. Magnolia can help with anxiety and depression. It contains magnolol and honokiol which are the active ingredients. Green tea on the other hand, has multiple benefits. It helps reduce anxiety via GABA receptors and contains catechins and proanthocyanidins as active ingredients. Because it contains caffeine it can interfere with sleep if taken too close to bedtime. It contains the amino acid **L-Theanine** which can be obtained as a separate supplement to aid sleep and anxiety. Green tea also has antioxidants that help prevent cell damage. It can help improve blood flow, reduce cardiovascular events, and improve memory. Green tea has also been shown to help block the formation of plaques that are associated with Alzheimer's disease. Green tea may also help blood sugar in diabetics, lower cholesterol, and lower blood pressure.

35. There are supplements that help with hot flashes, bone loss, and diabetes.

FOR HOT FLASHES

Valerian root will aid in the reduction of hot flashes along with phytoestrogens (which come from plants) such as **black cohosh**. It contains the active ingredient valerenic and also goes through the GABA receptors and glutamate receptors. It also helps reduce anxiety and has been used as a sleep aid.

FOR BONE LOSS

Red clover also contains phytoestrogens (which can help in menopausal symptoms) and recent studies have shown that it helps with bone mineralization. There were claims that it lowers cholesterol, but this is yet to be proven.

FOR DIABETES

Green tea, Berberine, Cinnamon, Chromium, Magnesium, and Vitamin D (only if deficient as it can be toxic at high levels) have been advocated for use in diabetics. Of questionable and unproven use

   WEIGHT LOSS *with* DIET EXERCISE STRESS REDUCTION

include aloe vera, bitter lemon, milk thistle, ginger, fenugreek, ginseng, and sweet potato.

FOR WEIGHT LOSS

36. There is no single supplement that will cause weight loss.

Most of the science journals will agree that no one supplement will help with weight loss. The combination of the DES principles and the supplements we advocate assist in promoting activities that will, in turn, help with weight loss. If we have a healthy microbiota, eat sensibly, develop good exercise habits, and learn to deal with our daily stress, weight loss will occur naturally.

37. Some supplements help joint pain, others that can help stimulate your natural growth hormone levels, and some that may help improve memory.

FOR MUSCLE
BUILDING AND STAMINA

Human growth hormone (HGH); The body produces this hormone naturally, but it decreases after you pass through puberty. It helps in muscle building, helps deep sleep, and fires up metabolism and libido. These benefits tend to gradually decrease as we age. You can, of course, inject synthetic HGH, but I would strongly argue against this. There are a few supplements you can take to stimulate your natural growth hormone. These are: **L arginine, L lysine, N-acetylcysteine,** and **L glutamine.**

FOR JOINT PAIN (INCLUDING RHEUMATOID ARTHRITIS)

L-Glutamine, curcumin, **Boswelia**, **GLA**, Magnesium citrate, and **methylated folic acid.** Boswelia is a tree native to India, Africa, and the Middle East. It is usually taken from the resin of the bark of the tree. It is believed that it acts as an anti-inflammatory. There have been some articles that suggest Boswellia may actually worsen autoimmune diseases such as rheumatoid arthritis, so use it with caution. Gamma linolenic acid (GLA) is an omega-6 fatty acid that is converted to other substances that the body uses to reduce inflammation. Evidence that this supplement is a benefit in rheumatoid arthritis is still questionable. Methylated folic acid can be used to improve gut health and is used to lower homocysteine levels. High homocysteine levels interfere with microcirculation including the blood vessels of the brain, gut, and joints. I would use this supplement only if you have high homocysteine levels.

FOR MEMORY

Supplements for memory are discussed later in the section on the DES diet and the brain. These supplements include **n-acetylcysteine** (NAC), a **multivitamin with minerals, omega-3,** and if deficient, **vitamin D.** You can add **methylated folic acid** if you have elevated homocysteine levels. **Curcumin** has also been associated with preserved cognition.

OTHER

For people that suffer from nausea and vomiting with their headaches, the addition of **thiamin** may be helpful.

L glutamine- We discussed this supplement earlier when discussing the microbiome. I will add that many times, it is also used for weight reduction, burning fat, and building muscle. That is why you will find this supplement in the Supermarket section for bodybuilding. It can also help boost your immune system.

If you have been paying attention you realize that L glutamine is very versatile and can be used for numerous functions. If you are to take only one supplement that would be the one. If you were to take two supplements, I would advise adding n-acetylcysteine which will help the immune system, memory, pulmonary expectorating function, is anti-cancer, anti-viral, anti-aging and has strong antioxidant function. Taking a multivitamin with minerals intermittently would be helpful, and the only other supplement would be the combination of arginine and lysine. These can also be taken intermittently. Omega 3 can be obtained by simply eating more fish. For now, take the supplements for gut health, especially during the cleanup period. **You must understand that almost half of the energy requirements of the gastrointestinal tract and liver are met with amino acids (protein) not just glucose.**

We should also note that several supplemental ingredients can potentially cause organ damage, cardiac arrest, and cancer. People with rheumatoid arthritis should avoid **aconite, arnica, arth-Q, cats' claw, chaparral**, and **Kombucha**. The biggest problem with most of these supplements is the amount. For instance, **caffeine powder** overdosing can cause heart arrhythmia, seizures, and possible cardiac arrest. **Coltsfoot** can produce liver damage, as can **usnic acid, red yeast rice, pennyroyal oil**, and **kava**. Coltsfoot is also a carcinogen. **Yohimbe** raises blood pressure and can produce headaches, heart problems, panic attacks, and liver problems. **Lobelia** can produce nausea, vomiting, diarrhea, and confusion. **Methylsynephrine** (the use is now illegal) can cause heart arrythmias especially when taken with other stimulants.

38. Many supplements are detrimental to your health especially when overdosing.

39. People with rheumatoid arthritis should be particularly careful with certain supplements which can actually cause more problems and worsen the disease.

We will soon be discussing the DES lifetime diet: Step Two. You will find yourself repeating the cleanup and cleansing diet several times a year. This will become evident as you start gaining weight, getting bloated, and begin to lose energy. An abbreviated two or three-day zero carbohydrate diet is usually enough to set the record straight again. Remember, we're balancing glycemic index, reduction of saturated fat and thus animal protein, and weight maintenance all at once. One type of diet cannot dominate the other.

THE REMAINING DIET-RELATED DES CONCEPTS ARE:

40. The Western diet is deficient in fiber and most people fail to consume the dietary minimum.

41. Try to balance the carbohydrate intake at approximately 30-35% of your total food consumption.

42. There are fiber supplements available but increase consumption gradually to avoid side effects.

43. Avoid large portions of the sweeter fruit.

44. The dirty dozen list represents fruits and vegetables high in pesticides and pesticide residues.

45. Wash, scrub, and rinse your fruit and vegetables before consuming.

46. Buy organic fruit and vegetables whenever possible.

 WEIGHT LOSS *with* DIET EXERCISE STRESS REDUCTION

47. Good hydration is important, but try not to overdo it to avoid water intoxication.

48. Depending on your activity level, consume two to five 8-ounce glasses of water daily.

49. Filtered water is preferable to tap water. Plastic water bottles should not be allowed to be exposed to high heat.

50. You obtain roughly half of your daily water requirements from the food you eat.

After you have completed the first week of the DES clean-up diet, carbohydrates can be reintroduced into the diet. We will allow you to select from the carbohydrate list below. These include the resistant starches discussed earlier. You want to maintain the carbohydrate percentage to one-third of your total caloric consumption. Normally, we were told to consume 40% of our diet as fat, 20% as protein, and 40% as carbohydrate. As discussed previously, this ratio changes as we enter a different stage in life. Young adults need more protein and as we age, we need less. People with diabetes, during diabetic diet counseling, are told to reduce carbohydrate consumption to only 25%. Unfortunately, our diets have been modified, and we tend to consume much more carbohydrates. This was particularly true when the so-called "experts" decided that we should not consume as much fat, which was substituted with carbs, and the low-fat diet fads began. Curiously, this is when the incidence of diabetes started to increase.

40. The Western diet is deficient in fiber and most people fail to consume the dietary minimum.

41. Try to balance the carbohydrate intake at approximately 30-35% of your total food consumption.

This list was prepared taking into consideration the fiber content of the fruits and vegetables. Men should consume 33–34 g of fiber daily, and women around 28 g of fiber. A typical Western diet provides only 18 g of daily fiber for men and 15 for women. I have been praising the accolades of a low-carb diet. Yet, I need to emphasize, you still need the carbohydrates, especially the high-fiber carbs.

There is a decrease in the incidence of cardiovascular disease mortality, stroke, and colon cancer with high-fiber diets. There is a decrease in weight and total cholesterol. The list of good carbs emphasizes the high fiber content and tends to be low in sugar. I tried to avoid the fruit issue as some are not as useful to the DES concepts as the ones on this list. Of course, you can have watermelon (high glycemic index), but keep in mind a pear will give you more fiber and less sugar.

FRUIT MOST HIGH IN FIBER:

- Figs
- Raspberries
- Pears
- Apple, with skin
- Blackberries
- Blueberries
- Mango
- Guava
- Prunes
- Orange
- Banana
- Strawberries

CEREALS:

- None of the sugary kind
- Psyllium
- Flaxseed
- Oats
- Bran flakes
- Brown rice
- Basmati rice
- Quinoa

BEANS (PREPARED IN THE PRESSURE COOKER IF LECTIN SENSITIVE)

- Lentils
- Chickpeas
- practically all the rest

VEGETABLES:

- Artichokes
- Peas
- Broccoli
- Avocado
- Acorn squash
- Edamame
- Collard greens
- Butternut squash
- Green bananas and plantain
- Cassava
- Olives
- Carrots

NUTS:

- Chia
- Pistachios
- Almonds
- Hemp
- Walnuts
- Pecans

OTHER:

- Popcorn
- Dark chocolate

Check the side panel and be cautious of the synthetic fibers, as their effect is unknown. These include cellulose, guar gum, and intrinsic plant fibers. I am always concerned about non-digestible fiber. You can also add a fiber supplement to your diet. A high-fiber diet can give you gas and bloating if you are not used to it. Go slow when adding new high-fiber fruit and vegetables.

42. There are fiber supplements available but increase consumption gradually to avoid side effects.

FRUIT

43. Avoid large portions of the sweeter fruit.

Fructose is a natural sugar. It is a carbohydrate which means it needs to be consumed with care. Fruit is an excellent source of fiber, and it has a relatively low glycemic index as it must be metabolized into glucose prior to utilization. During the cleanup part of the DES diet, we ask you not to eat any fruit, but after the first week, fruit can be added. I would still **avoid large portions** of the sweeter fruit which include:

- Apricots
- Mangos
- Melon
- Pineapple
- Papaya
- Plums
- Prunes

Eating too much fruit may trigger sugar addiction again and sabotage our efforts to clean the gut. Berries are the best choice. They have good amounts of antioxidants and fiber.

WEIGHT LOSS *with* DIET EXERCISE STRESS REDUCTION

THE DIRTY DOZEN

44. The dirty dozen list represents fruits and vegetables high in pesticides and pesticide residues.

I really do not want to complicate the diet concepts any more than they already are, but the dirty dozen merits mentioning. This list represents foods that are high in pesticides. The list is put out by the Environmental Working Group (EWG). It is a list of pesticide residues in non-organic fruits and vegetables. We have already mentioned the negative effects of pesticides on our health. By following the DES diet, you will be consuming greater amounts of fruit and vegetables to feel healthier. Loading up on more pesticide residue does not seem to be a good idea. We will thus present you with the dirty dozen:

1.   Strawberries (over ten pesticide residues)
2.   Spinach (high in permethrin, a neurotoxin)
3.   Nectarines (over 15 different pesticide residues)
4.   Apples (90% of samples contained pesticide residues)
5.   Grapes (96% contained residues)
6.   Peaches (99% contained residues)
7.   Cherries
8.   Pears
9.   Tomatoes
10. Celery
11. Potatoes (contained more residues by weight than any other crop)
12. Sweet bell peppers (may contain less residues, but those present are more toxic)

There are a few more that should be mentioned as well: blueberries, hot peppers, cherry tomatoes, and snap peas.

There are some methods you can use to reduce the amount of pesticide residues on your produce. Apples can be washed in 1% baking soda solution. Peeling, blanching, and boiling can reduce the residues. Scrubbing and rinsing your fruit and vegetables can also reduce the pesticide residues. Buy organic if possible. Granted, they are more expensive, but they may be worth it in the end. You can also start an herb and vegetable garden. You can be certain it is organic; you grew it yourself!

45. Wash, scrub, and rinse your fruit and vegetables before consuming.

46. Buy organic fruit and vegetables whenever possible.

WATER

47. Good hydration is important but try not to overdo it to avoid water intoxication.

48. Depending on your activity level, consume two to five eight-ounce glasses of water daily.

Water consumption should not be a controversial subject, but somehow it has become one. Some experts say to drink eight glasses of water a day. In contrast, others say to drink when you are thirsty. Every other expert will recommend some in between number of glasses of water a day. Who do we believe? The body maintains its electrolyte balance during the day and when exercising. When there is not enough water the body excretes more salt from the kidneys and sweat to maintain this balance. So, for the most part it is usually unnecessary to supplement with electrolytes before a workout. Ben Greenfield states "You should simply drink when you are thirsty." Dr. Gundry recommends drinking 8 to 10 glasses of water daily. Dr. Perlmutter recommends keeping water with you all the time. His only

   WEIGHT LOSS *with* DIET EXERCISE STRESS REDUCTION

other recommendation is that we use filtered water, I agree. So, let us break down the fluid intake and output. In 24 hours, insensible water loss through the skin is approximately 400 mL (13 ½ ounces). Insensible water loss through the respiratory tract is an additional 400 mL. Insensible water loss is defined as water loss that you cannot control. On the other hand, you actually produce water through metabolic processes which amounts to about 400 mL a day. In order to produce urine, you need a minimum of 500 mL of water a day. Sweating usually produces 100 mL of fluid loss and we lose an additional 200 mL through feces. This total amounts to 1600 mL of water loss daily (54 ounces) **minimum**. This is then contrasted with the intake. It is estimated that half your fluid intake is supplied in the food we eat (800 mL). We also have to account for water produced through metabolism, which is 400 mL, which leaves a minimal amount of 400 mL to 600 mL (13.5 oz-20 oz). This translates into one and one-half 8-ounce glass of water to almost three 8-ounce glasses of water daily. Since this is the minimum, and with the DES concepts, you are expected to sweat, drinking anywhere from 4 to 8 glasses of water a day would be adequate. I also believe in drinking only when you are thirsty. You can also let your urine color be your guide; if it is too dark, drink up. You need to replace 32 ounces of water for every hour of sweating activity in which you engage (80-degree heat, 80% humidity one hour from the moment you start sweating).

49. Filtered water is preferable to tap water. Plastic water bottles should not be allowed to be exposed to high heat.

50. You obtain roughly half of your daily water requirement from the food you eat.

The DES concepts that follow are related to exercise. These include:

51. We need to maintain muscle tone and mass by using them.

52. Get medical clearance before you start a vigorous exercise program and start slow.

53. Get some daily physical activity even if it is just for 10 to 15 minutes.

54. Any amount of exercise is beneficial, cardio exercise is even better.

55. Three hours of aerobic exercise a week increased life expectancy by approximately ten years.

56. Walking will burn 314 calories an hour.

57. Running more than 20 miles (32.2 km) a week begins to undo the cardiovascular benefits of running.

58. Some sport watches can help count steps, monitor your sleep, and even tell you recovery time needed after you work out.

59. Running shoes need to be replaced about every 300 miles (483 km) as they tend to lose their resiliency.

60. Do not be afraid to sweat.

61. A sports watch may be helpful to keep track of your heart rate so that your pulse will remain at no more than 80% maximum for your age when you first start an exercise program.

62. Aerobic exercise can lower cholesterol, raise HDL, help with weight maintenance, and decrease anxiety and depression.

63. It is important to maintain an exercise regimen not just for a few weeks, but for the rest of your life.

64. Although not for everyone, going to the gym can motivate you to exercise.

65. There are other ways of toning muscle other than weightlifting.

66. Resistance exercises have many advantages that can help you maintain body weight and muscle tone and save time, especially with our busy schedules.

EXERCISE

The second point of our triangle is exercise. It has been confirmed that any amount of exercise is superior to no exercise. As we get older, we contend with deconditioning, when we become less active. In addition to this, we must deal with sarcopenia, which is the loss of muscle mass in men and women. Our muscles gradually substitute fat for muscle fibers, and subsequently, we become weaker and lose muscle mass. After the age of 40 you potentially lose ten percent muscle mass per decade. To counteract this phenomenon, we must maintain good muscle tone by way of exercise. It is no wonder that people who remain physically active in their middle age and into their 50s and 60s go on to live well into their 80s. It is one thing to make it to 90 in a wheelchair than make it to 90 walking to the plaza! If you are not physically active or have a medical condition, you may need to talk to your doctor to learn which activities are safe for you. Find the physical activity that you can enjoy and keep with over time. Get some form of physical activity every day, **even if it is just 10-15 minutes**. Make it a routine. Start with a small amount of exercise and increase the time.

Park further away from the store or take a walk around the block. Move at a pace that feels right for you and increase the cadence as you get used to it. Work towards eventually choosing several types of cardiovascular and muscle strengthening activities. The goal is 150 minutes of moderate physical activity per week.

51. We need to maintain muscle tone and mass by using them.

52. Get medical clearance before you start a vigorous exercise program and start slow.

53. Get some physical activity every day, even if for only 10-15 minutes.

I feel that trying to reach the age of 110 is not really a feasible goal for most of us (it occurs to one in 3 million people). Still, our goal should be to become a super-senior. These individuals are in their 80s and are as active as 35-year-olds. So, when do we begin an exercise program? The answer is easy: right now. Maintain good muscle tone by lifting light weights, going up stairs, when possible, push-ups, sit-ups, calisthenics, walking, running, playing team sports, etc. The easiest of all is walking. If you add running at intervals, we are then really doing the body good. There have been studies that demonstrated increased longevity in individuals who performed aerobic exercise (cardio). Aerobic exercise added an average of ten years increased in life expectancy in those who exercised three hours or more a week. Those individuals who exercised two hours a week had an increase in life expectancy of 5 to 6 years. Those who had one hour of aerobic exercise a week increased their life expectancy by 2 to 3 years over those who did not exercise at all.

54. Any amount of exercise is beneficial; cardio exercise is even better.

55. Three hours of aerobic exercise a week increases life expectancy by ten years.

SELECT YOUR EXERCISE

Caloric expenditure for exercise will vary depending on the type of exercise you are performing. On average, walking will burn 314 calories per hour of exercise. Running 5 miles an hour will burn 606 calories per hour. Low impact aerobic exercise will burn 365 calories an hour while water aerobics can burn 402 calories. Using an elliptical trainer at moderate effort will burn 365 calories per hour and golfing while carrying your clubs could burn 314. Swimming laps with light or moderate effort will burn 423 calories. Bicycling at less than 10 mph will burn 292 calories per hour. Notice that walking burns more calories than leisurely riding a bike.

56. Walking will burn 314 calories an hour.

RUNNING

There was a point in my life where I believed that the secret to longevity and health was running. I was an avid runner, running 15 to 20 miles a week. At times, I would run 24 to 25 miles per week and saw an article that suggested a detrimental effect of long-distance running. This would be a good time to discuss that " U " shaped curve. The top of the " U " is a parameter that is modified by a factor. At the base are the miles run per week and the parameter we are measuring is that of the risk cardiovascular events. As we increase the miles run per week, we start the downslope of the " U " (less risk) and reach a nadir in which the maximum benefit has been reached. As we increase the miles ran per week, we go on the upslope of the " U, " the beneficial effect starts fading to a point where we reach no beneficial effect at all! It is the proverbial too much of a good thing is bad for you. So, you are wondering, at what point does the curve start rising again? It is 20 miles per week. More than that, you start undoing the benefits and you also risk wear- and- tear on your joints and other injuries.

Since any exercise is better than no exercise, I recommend that each of you select whatever exercise regimen you would like.

57. Running more than 20 miles (32.2 km) a week begins to undo the cardiovascular benefits of running.

This would be a good time to tell the story of Pheidippides. He was a professional courier for the Greek army that had just succeeded in defeating the Persians at the Battle of Marathon. He ran approximately 25 miles to Athens and was able to relay the good news of the victory. He died upon stating "Victory!". This is now known as Pheidippides cardiomyopathy. The stresses of long-distance running will take a toll on the heart. It is well known that cardiac enzymes (a measure of heart muscle destruction) will rise in marathoners. The theory is that constant stress on the heart will lead to scarring of the cardiac muscle and eventually to cardiac arrhythmias.

58. Some sport watches can help count steps, monitor your sleep, and even tell you recovery time needed after your workout.

59. Running shoes need to be replaced at around 300-350 miles (483-563 km) and at times sooner depending on how you run.

You should note that after a certain number of miles, usually around 300 miles (483 km), the shoes lose their resiliency, bounce, and are too loose. This is particularly true when using them for running. Shoes also come for neutral, underpronator, and overpronator stride. You may be a heel, mid-foot, or toe striker. You can actually change the step strike by changing the positioning of your hands. There is a reflex positioning of the feet in response to the positioning of your hands and wrist. My research failed to reveal a name for this phenomenon, so I call it the Berrios reflex. Your feet will pronate if you pronate your hand and wrist (palms down), making you strike more over the arch, or if you supinate your hand and

   WEIGHT LOSS *with* DIET EXERCISE STRESS REDUCTION

wrist (palms up) you will strike towards the edge of your foot. Likewise, flexing your hand and wrist will make you strike over your heels, and extending your wrist will make you strike over your toes. This information may be helpful if you sustain injuries or have tender feet or ankles so you can modify your strike point.

WALKING

Several different exercises can be performed to maintain our physical fitness, and the most popular is walking. Walking is the most basic form of exercise that will help us give up sedentary lifestyles. Aside from the previously mentioned health benefits, it will lead to lower body mass indexes, trimmer waists, and better scores on measures of heart disease and diabetes. But it would be nice to determine what would be the best stride for you. It helps to count your steps, which is where the smartwatch can help as it will count them for you. If you are a slow walker you may want to pick up the pace just a bit. If you are a fast walker, then increase your pace even further; just make it a little more than your normal pace. You may want to join a group or invite a friend to walk with you. Stretches of inactivity are detrimental to our health, so fill your day with short walks. Use the stairs when possible.

The usual safety precautions merit mentioning. Wear sunscreen to protect the skin from skin cancer, but not too much or cover too much of the body as you still want to activate Vitamin D. Sunscreen will help, but so will sunshades. UV light is a common cause of cataracts in the elderly. You must sweat! Sweat not only cools the body but also serves as another venue to rid our bodies of toxins. Other advice would follow logic as we would need comfortable shoes, loose-fitting clothing and clothing designed for exercising. And why not look good in the process? You need to walk in areas in which there is low vehicular traffic, and even walking trails, so as not to cause injury or falls.

Step counting is a popular approach to providing physical activity. An optimal dose of 6,000 to 8,000 steps has been suggested to reduce the risk of all-cause mortality. Higher step counts may lower the risk of heart disease and cancer. They may even reduce the incidence of diabetes, especially with higher intensity walking. A recent study in the UK suggested that approximately 9,800 steps per day may be optimal to lower the risk of dementia. They estimated that the minimum dose was approximately 3,800 steps per day, which is associated with a 25% lower incidence of dementia. Previous studies have been directed to investigate mortality outcomes. This particular study was directed at correlating with dementia outcomes.

60. Do not be afraid to sweat.

61. A sports watch may be helpful to keep track of your heart rate so that your pulse will remain at no more than 80% of the maximum for your age when first starting an exercise program.

Most of this advice has been directed to individuals in their 40s and 50s who are still in some degree of good physical shape. But what if you are in your 60s and you have neglected your body, not only by eating the wrong food, but also by being inactive and deconditioned? For those starting, I will recommend a few other modifications. I strongly recommend obtaining a sports watch that can keep track of your heart rate. Some can be quite cumbersome as they require a chest band. The more expensive watches can provide heart rate as long as you do not sweat too much (and I want you to!). A wrist sweatband will sometimes cut down on the wrist sweat and allow the watch to provide adequate heart rate data. I have noticed a recent improvement in sweat resistance of the newer watches. It can be somewhat of a problem to program the watch. Still, it is quite rewarding as you need to know if you are approaching maximum exercise tolerance. If you are totally deconditioned, we strongly recommend that you start slow, as we are in no hurry. You have had weight loss by modifying your diet, so do not go out and try to run a marathon the first time you exercise. I do not want you to take your heart rate to the limit (100%) but rather take it to 70% and max out at 80%. The watch usually calculates your maximum heart rate by subtracting your age from 220 beats per minute. If not, you could do that yourself and subsequently calculate 90%, 80%, 70%, etc.

If your pulse rate does not increase very much just by walking, then you can add running at intervals. Say every three 10ths of a mile, you can run a 10th of a mile. On the contrary if your pulse rate goes up too fast because you are not used to exercising, you must know when you have reached your pulse rate goal so you can rest. The newer GPS watches will not only give you your pulse rate but will also give you your distance so you can calculate the distance you can walk-run. They can be a useful tool and can not only tell you how many miles you are running a week, but also where you ran them, which can be quite useful when going on vacations. You will have a record of every place you ran or walked and a record for an entire year. It can tell you how many steps you've taken, which can also motivate you to walk more, and even keep track of how many miles you have walked or run in a pair of shoes.

62. Aerobic exercise can lower cholesterol, raise HDL, help with weight maintenance, and decrease anxiety and depression.

63. It is important to maintain an exercise regimen, not just for a few weeks, but for the rest of your life.

What are the cardiovascular benefits of cardio exercise? There are several. It can help lower cholesterol and blood pressure. It can help you lose weight coupled with a reasonable diet. Exercise increases your good cholesterol (HDL), and similarly the beneficial effect disappears if you stop exercising for just six weeks. So, it is very important to maintain an exercise regimen, not just for a few weeks but **for the rest of your life.** One of the most beneficial effects of cardio exercise is the recent discovery that three hours of cardio exercise a week resulted in a reduction of anxiety and depressive symptoms in affected subjects by approximately 60%!

HITTING THE GYM

64. Although it is not for everyone, going to the gym can motivate you to exercise.

65. There are other ways of toning muscle other than weightlifting.

66. Resistance exercises have many advantages that can help you maintain body weight and muscle tone, and save time, especially with our busy schedules.

The gym is like the candy store to the kid: so many choices that they cannot make up their minds. Do I do the elliptical? Should I hit the treadmill? Should I go swimming? To wade through these choices, you may want to seek the help of a professional personal trainer. The truth is any type of exercise will be beneficial to the body; you do not need to turn into a well-tuned athlete to reap the benefits of exercise. The gym is excellent for strength training. We had mentioned earlier about losing muscle mass as we age. This will happen even if we stay fit. You can learn to lift weights and tune up the muscles. Just remember to perform aerobic activity (cardio) and use muscle strengthening for the major muscle groups in the proportion you can handle. There are other ways of strengthening your muscles without lifting weights. You can use resistance bands which come in different tension levels and offer one of the safest weight-bearing workouts. You can use the machines at the gym that load different muscles and do not require picking up a weight or loading a bar. Another way of exercise includes performing squats, lunges, or push-ups. Some workouts can include isometric exercises or even yoga which uses your body weight as resistance.

      WEIGHT LOSS *with* DIET EXERCISE STRESS REDUCTION

RESISTANCE TRAINING

Resistance training is a form of exercise. As the name suggests, it involves exercising muscles using some form of resistance. This will help increase muscular strength, endurance, and is associated with better sleep. The resistance could be weights, bands, or even your body weight working against gravity. It is sometimes called strength training or weight training. The Centers for Disease Control and Prevention recommends performing muscle strengthening exercises and activities of moderate or greater intensity approximately two to four days a week. Studies have found that resistance exercises can boost your metabolism and help in weight loss. Resistance training exercise can reduce menopausal hot flashes. Some studies actually indicated that resistance training was more effective for improving your metabolism than aerobic exercise. Rather than compete with aerobic exercise, these exercise programs tend to supplement each other and should be part of your routine. Since we do not perform aerobic exercise every day, on the days you don't, you can perform resistance exercises, including push-ups, pull-ups, kettlebells, dumbbells, stretch bands, etc.

A recent study found that a combination of aerobic and strength exercises was additive and increased life expectancy even more than each alone.

The following DES concepts relate to stress. I have also included some concepts related to sleep:

67. Stress can harm the body and mind. It can be the harbinger of disease.

68. We need to identify the sources of stress in our lives in order to deal with them and eventually reduce the negative effects they could have on our lives.

69. Biofeedback can be a tool in reducing stress.

70. Do not underestimate the power of prayer in reducing stress and helping us cope with stressful situations.

71. Tai chi and yoga are helpful in reducing stress and keeping us fit.

72. Mindfulness techniques can provide health benefits.

73. Breathing exercises can help reduce stress and are easy to do.

74. Sleep apnea can cause daytime sleepiness, fatigue, memory problems, depression, and decreased libido and can be treated with weight loss.

75. Good quality sleep is essential for normal body and mind functioning.

76. Exposure to light can affect sleep patterns dramatically.

77. Excessive use of tablets and smartphones can disrupt sleep and cause delayed sleep phase.

78. Sleep helps rid the brain of toxins.

79. Follow good sleep hygiene principles to obtain good quality sleep.

STRESS REDUCTION

67. Stress can harm the body and mind. It can be the harbinger of disease.

Stress is a silent killer that can have devastating effects on both physical and mental health. Psychological stress has been known to increase the risk of heart attacks and stroke. It has been correlated with actual structural brain changes that can be seen on MRI scans. In today's fast-paced world, we are constantly bombarded with demands from work, family, and social obligations, leaving us feeling overwhelmed and stressed. The long-term effects of stress can shorten life expectancy and affect our emotional well-being.

We need to approach stress management by first identifying the specific stressors in life. Once you have identified the stressors, you can attempt to eliminate them and if they cannot be eliminated, then be able to cope and function despite the stressors. There are several ways of keeping calm. Breathing is one of the most accessible and easiest ways to calm the nervous system in any situation. One of the easiest ways is to take a long deep breath into your stomach, allowing your belly to expand. You can fold your hands over your belly and see them rise. Follow a simple four-step breath work process as follows:

1. Breathe in for a count of four seconds.

2. Hold your breath for a count of four seconds.

3. Breathe out for a count of four seconds.

4. Hold your breath for a count of four seconds.

You can continue this process for as long as you need, and you should begin to feel calm within a couple of repetitions. This is known as box breathing. Box breathing is also called "tactical breathing" and is used by the US military as a way of stress management. Other breathing techniques include: circular breathing which involves taking long, slow breaths filling and emptying the lungs without pausing between breaths; conscious connected breathing that includes a period of rest between long inhalations and exhalations; and cyclic sighing, in which the exhalations are sustained longer than the inhalations.

Spending time with nature is another effective way to reduce stress. Studies have found that **just 20 minutes in nature soothes the nervous system** and can help us feel relaxed. Whether it is going for a walk in the park, hiking in the mountains, or simply sitting in a quiet place surrounded by greenery, spending time in nature can provide us with much-needed respite from the stressors of daily life.

WEIGHT LOSS *with* DIET EXERCISE STRESS REDUCTION

SPIRE STONE™ FITBIT CHARGE ™ APPLE WATCH ™ GARMIN WATCHES ™

Identify your enemy. There are many stressors in our lives of which we are not aware. One technological gadget that can help identify these stressors is one that would monitor respirations. I will mention two of these, but there are others. The respiratory rate increases as we become more stressed. One such device is Spire. Spire is a small gadget that you wear on the body to monitor respiratory rates. It is coupled to your smart phone and will tell you when your respiratory rate increases (stressed). By knowing when this occurs you can attempt to abort the stressful situation by meditation and other relaxation techniques. The app itself will tell you to take a rest and will guide you through breathing exercises. Another gadget that could also serve as an activity tracker is the Fitbit Charge. This one has the added advantage of having a daily Stress Management Score showing your body's response to stress. Apple watches and certain Garmin watches can also guide you to breathing exercises and are very convenient. Once you identify a specific stressor, you can then attempt to modify or eliminate it. Unfortunately, many of the stressors cannot be eliminated and we must decide how to cope with them. We will discuss these techniques.

68. We need to identify the sources of stress in our lives in order to deal with them and eventually reduce the negative effects they could have on our lives.

BIOFEEDBACK

69. Biofeedback can be a tool in reducing stress.

Biofeedback is defined as a technique to gain control over normally involuntary functions. It has been used to reduce pain and decades ago it was used as a treatment for migraine headaches. It can also be used for incontinence and high blood pressure. With biofeedback techniques you are trying to harness the power of your mind and become aware of what is going on inside your body and autonomic nervous system. For example, one such technique used for migraine treatment was to allow the subject to hold a skin temperature thermometer and watch as the temperature of the skin increases. This would allow for vasodilation of the blood vessels in the hands diverting blood away from the brain and scalp. This in turn would result in a reduction in the throbbing pain of the headache. Other biofeedback techniques include monitoring of the brain waves and allowing the person to visualize them on a monitor screen. The idea is for the person to become relaxed enough so he or she can see their alpha waves dominate the electrographic record. Neuroscientists have created miniature trains that will be powered on only if the person is in alpha state (relaxed). You can also monitor heart rate, which is probably the easiest to master. By utilizing other techniques such as meditation and breathing exercises the person receives biofeedback information in the form of a slowing of the heart rate which he or she can monitor. A smart watch can display a constant heart rate reading and would be helpful for this.

MEDITATION AND PRAYER

Meditation is a powerful tool that can help with stress and improve our overall health and well-being. Meditation has been shown to reduce the decline of gray matter in the brain as well as help us deal with pain and anxiety. There are many different types of meditation, each with its unique approach and benefits. Some of the most popular types of meditation include mindful meditation, transcendental meditation (TM), analytical meditation, breath meditation, and Vipassana meditation.

    WEIGHT LOSS *with* DIET EXERCISE STRESS REDUCTION

It is important to note that prayer can also produce benefits similar to meditation. Studies have shown that people of faith live longer. By focusing on a higher power and connecting with a sense of purpose, prayer can help us reduce stress and improve our overall physical and mental health.

Mindful meditation involves becoming aware of your present-moment experiences and observing them without judgment. This type of meditation encourages you to focus on your thoughts, emotions, and physical sensations and learn to accept them as they are. By doing so, you are able to develop greater awareness and clarity, and you are able to cultivate a more peaceful and mindful approach to life.

Transcendental meditation (TM) is a simple, effortless technique that involves repeating a mantra of sound in your mind. This type of meditation is designed to help you reach a state of deep relaxation and inner peace. By focusing on the mantra, you are able to let go of distracting thoughts and emotions, allowing your mind to settle into a state of stillness and calm. This meditation is good for calming the mind.

Analytical meditation involves exploring your thoughts and emotions in a non-judgmental way. This type of meditation encourages you to observe your thoughts and emotions objectively as they arise without getting caught up or attached to them. By doing so, you are able to gain greater insight into your mental and emotional states and develop a more detached and peaceful relationship with your thoughts and emotions.

Breath meditation is another popular type of meditation that involves focusing on your breath. By paying close attention to the sensation of your breath as it moves in and out of your body, you are able to quiet your mind and reduce stress. This type of meditation can be especially helpful for those who struggle with anxiety or sleep issues, as it can help calm the nervous system and promote a sense of relaxation and peace.

A more demanding and extreme form of meditation is Vipassana meditation. It is a type of meditation that is particularly effective in reducing stress and improving mental health. This type of meditation is focused on developing awareness of our physical sensations and learning to observe them so we can deal with them in a nonreactive manner. By doing so, Vipassana meditation helps to strengthen our minds and cope with stress by dealing with the sensations in the body. This type of meditation is effective because it helps us become aware of the underlying causes of our stress and develop the skills to manage it in a healthy, effective way.

We have described different types of meditation, each with his own unique approach benefit. Whether you choose mindful meditation, Transcendental meditation, or any of the other types of meditation, taking the time to meditate can help you reduce stress and improve your health, cultivate greater peace, and create mental wellness.

70. Do not underestimate the power of prayer in reducing stress and helping us cope with stressful situations.

TAI CHI AND YOGA

Tai Chi is particularly effective in reducing stress and anxiety, as the slow, controlled movements coupled with deep breathing help to calm the mind and promote relaxation. This technique is sometimes called "meditation in motion." In addition to reducing stress, Tai Chi can improve flexibility, increase muscle strength and definition, and enhance overall physical health. This is particularly important for older adults as Tai Chi has been shown to help maintain balance and reduce the risk of falls. Similarly, yoga is also known for stress-reducing and calming effects. Like Tai Chi, yoga can improve flexibility, muscle strength, and overall physical health. Tai Chi and yoga have been shown to help with chronic low back pain and even help reduce menstrual pain. However, yoga is also known for its mental benefits as the practice of focusing on the breath and body can help to quiet the mind and promote inner peace. In addition to traditional forms of Tai Chi and yoga, there are newer variations and styles to choose from, including styles that focus on specific areas of the body or mental states. For example, yoga with goats is a newer and growing

  WEIGHT LOSS *with* DIET EXERCISE STRESS REDUCTION

trend where participants practice yoga surrounded by goats! This style of yoga is designed to be fun and playful. It is a great way to bring a sense of lightheartedness to the practice of yoga, although it can be very distracting.

Tai chi and yoga are both powerful practices that offer a range of physical and mental benefits. Whether you are looking to reduce stress, improve physical health, or simply try to find a new form of exercise, Tai Chi and yoga are both worth considering.

71. Tai Chi and yoga are helpful in reducing stress and keeping us fit.

72. Mindfulness techniques can provide health benefits.

73. Breathing exercises can help reduce stress and are easy to do.

If you are looking to further explore mindfulness, relaxation techniques, and exercise programs there are many resources available to you including books, YouTube videos, and in-person courses. There are many streaming services available for yoga, meditation, and exercise. Here are some options to consider:

1. **DOWN DOG:** This app offers a range of yoga classes for different levels and styles as well as customizable workouts for strength training and HIIT (high intensity interval training).

2. **PELOTON DIGITAL:** This app offers a variety of classes, including yoga, strength training and meditation led by certified instructors.

3. **HEADSPACE:** Headspace offers guided meditations, mindfulness sessions, and sleep aids to help you relax and reduce stress.

4. **GLO:** Glo features yoga, meditation, and Pilates classes taught by renowned instructors from around the world.

5. **FIT ON**: This app offers a mix of yoga, Pilates, HIIT, and other workouts led by certified trainers.

6. **GAIA**: This app offers a variety of yoga and meditation classes as well as documentaries and interviews with experts in the wellness world.

7. **SWEAT COIN**: With this app you receive rewards for staying active. The app uses the phone's GPS and motion sent to track activities like walking, running, and cycling. It converts it into a currency called sweat coins. Users can spend their sweat coins on various products and services that are offered by the app's partners including wellness products, fitness gear, and even vacations. It aims to incentivize healthy behavior and encourage people to stay active by offering tangible rewards for their efforts.

We have just scratched the surface of the available apps on the Internet and streaming options. It is worth your while to explore different options and select one that suits your needs and preferences.

Now that you understand the concepts for the DES clean-up diet, the need for exercise and the role of stress reduction we will provide the main changes you need to make.

PUTTING IT ALL TOGETHER:

DES CONCEPTS STEP ONE

DIET

- You will consume only vegetables and meat for one week.
- You will not consume any fruit during this week, but you can consume **dairy, eggs,** and **soy products**.
- You cannot consume sodas.
- Eliminate all desserts.
- Eliminate all inflammatory foods (page 12).
- Eliminate all ultra-processed foods (page 18).
- Eliminate all alcohol (or limit to one ounce or less a day) and all fruit juices.
- Consume only two meals a day, a brunch at around 11:30 in the morning and dinner from 6 to 7pm.

If you do snack, do so midafternoon and before bedtime. Make it less than 200 calories and make it your favorite nut. Yogurt (unsweetened), avocado, popcorn without sugar, and hard cheese are also acceptable. Nothing with high sugar content or starch.

Start L-glutamine 2000 mg daily with a meal the week before and during the clean-up diet then 1000 mg daily thereafter.

Be aware that you can suffer from hypoglycemia when starting this diet.

EXERCISE

DURING THE STEP ONE DIET WEEK:

You will walk one mile three times for that week. Do not make it a leisurely walk. Instead, try for a 16–17-minute mile. Okay, 18 minutes is still good. Too busy and have no time? You can walk 1 ½ miles twice that week on Saturday and Sunday. Perform squats, pushups, lunges, or whatever resistance exercise you choose on two non-walking days.

STRESS REDUCTION

Breathing exercises should be performed daily. This is particularly true during stressful situations. It is also a good way to start your day. You will start with the 3/3/3/3 pattern. Breathe in for three seconds, hold for three, then exhale for three seconds, then hold for three. Do this for two or three minutes.

DES CONCEPTS STEP TWO

DIET

You will forever eliminate sodas, fruit juices, seed oils, desserts, and ultra processed and inflammatory foods.

Reintroduce the carbohydrates and these will now be of low glycemic index, low glycemic load, resistant starches, and high fiber.

EXERCISE

DURING STEP TWO OF THE DIET:

You will walk two miles twice a week forever. As it becomes a habit you can add running for short distances to get the pulse rate up a little. If you are still motivated, then increase to three times a week. Continue to perform resistance exercises twice a week.

STRESS REDUCTION

Once a day attempt to dedicate 5 minutes to the 4/4/4/4 breathing exercise. Just like the three-second exercise, you will instead perform the exercise in four-second intervals. By this time, you have selected a relaxation technique to try. Join a yoga class (with or without goats!), a gym, a cycling group, a spin class, etc. Stay with it forever. This will be the same for Step Three (page 67).

SLEEP

Most of us are aware of the importance of sleep. We all sleep, but it does not guarantee an understanding of its complexities. We all need sleep. There is a pleasurable feeling to hit the pillow when we are sleepy and sleep without any problem. Then to awaken rested, clear-headed, and energetic. Many times, that is not the case, with poor sleep often leading to daytime drowsiness.

In the elderly, poor sleep may be the result of chronic pain, sleep apnea, or due to medication side effects. The use of sleeping pills tends to increase with age, and elderly women are proportionately higher users of sedative hypnotic products than elderly men. Daytime sleepiness because of inadequate sleep has been linked to 20% to 25% of car accidents, highlighting its significance.

Your sleep drive is dictated by the amount of sleep you had the 24 hours prior. As we age, our sleep requirements decrease. Adults after the age of 65 may need as little as 5 to 6 hours of sleep as reported by the National Sleep

Foundation. However, sleep loss does not cause irreversible brain damage. The effects of acute or chronic sleep loss are fully reversible. Researchers have found that human beings can go without sleep for as long as 36 hours with no significant physical or psychological consequences.

Even healthy individuals occasionally experience difficulty falling asleep or have restless sleep. Sometimes, they sleep but awaken tired and still groggy, while others struggle with sleep on a nightly basis. We do have medical terms for these situations. Insomnia of sleep onset (getting to sleep), sleep maintenance (not staying asleep), and sleep conditions that manifest as excessive daytime sleepiness. Sleep and health go hand-in-hand. Poor sleep can affect your health, and poor health can affect your sleep. The aim of the DES concepts is not to diagnose or treat medical conditions, but rather to promote natural sleep through sensible eating, exercise, and stress management.

SLEEP APNEA

Although the DES concepts do not directly address sleep-related diseases, they can indirectly influence them. Sleep apnea is a process in which nocturnal ventilation is compromised. Apnea in Latin means "without air". The usual cause of sleep apnea is a total blockage or partial blockage (hypopnea) of the airway, obstructing the flow of air into the lungs. The blockage can occur at the level of the nose, the back of the throat or at the base of the tongue. When we sleep, the muscles in the throat and pharynx relax and the tissues collapse upon themselves, closing the airway. The resultant lack of oxygen will continuously awaken the person in order to take a breath. These arousals are too short for the person to notice but can disrupt the continuity of sleep so much as to cause daytime symptoms. These can include sleepiness, fatigue, slow thinking process, depression, and even lack of sexual drive. The lack of oxygen is not as common but, in more severe cases, will contribute to daytime sleepiness, fatigue, and mood changes. While following the DES concepts cannot directly address

  WEIGHT LOSS *with* DIET EXERCISE STRESS REDUCTION

airway blockage, weight loss achieved through following these concepts can help alleviate symptoms. Other conventional treatments include not only weight loss, but mandibular advancement devices that move the jaw forward, allowing more air to flow at the base of the tongue. It may also include continuous positive airway pressure (CPAP), which is a mechanical blower forcing air into the nose and at times the mouth at a set pressure; this acts to keep the airway open. Nasal sprays can help keep the nasal passages open, and sleeping on your side can help move air easier.

74. Sleep apnea can cause daytime sleepiness, fatigue, memory problems, depression and low libido and can improve with weight loss.

It should also be noted that certain medications will worsen sleep apnea. These are: sodium oxybate (Xyrem), Rofecoxib (Vioxx), Alendronic acid (Fosamax, Binostro), Digoxin, Quetiapine, esomeprazole (Nexium) and Clozapine (Clozaril).

I have made a list of symptoms related to sleep apnea (compromised breathing during sleep). You may not notice the symptoms yourself, but rather a family member or bed partner may have commented on them. These symptoms are:

1. **SNORING:** It is the most common symptom and most noticeable by the bed partner. It may be associated with snorting and interrupted by silences. An explosive, expiratory reprise may sometimes be present.

2. **ABNORMAL MOTOR MOVEMENTS DURING SLEEP:** There is increased tossing and turning during the night. It may range from simple movements of the extremities to large movements of the arms and legs, causing unwitting slaps or kicks to the bed partner. If there is a significant drop in oxygen during the night, a large movement of the upper part of the body may be seen, which leads to a half-seated position followed by a drop of the head back to the pillow.

3. **NOCTURNAL SLEEP INTERRUPTIONS:** People may awaken from sleep numerous times during the night because of difficulty breathing due to sleep apnea. They are unaware of the frequency and intensity of the disruptive sleep pattern during the night and will complain of insomnia.

4. **HEARTBURN:** When the airway is obstructed, there is an increase in esophageal and gastric pressures. These can produce acid reflux.

5. **URINATING AT NIGHT:** It is thought that the increase in abdominal pressure associated with respiratory efforts exerts pressure on the bladder. Abnormal sleep patterns and awakening confusion have also been associated.

6. **CHOKING:** Some people feel like they are choking or gagging when awakening in the middle of the night. They may even get up and run to a window, trying to take a deep breath.

7. **SWEATING:** Excessive movements and sleep restlessness can cause this symptom.

8. **SLEEPINESS DURING THE DAY:** Although this is a subjective complaint, if you fall asleep at inappropriate times, such as driving, watching television, or reading a book, it could be a sign of disrupted nocturnal sleep.

9. **HEADACHES:** This can occur due to low oxygen or excessive carbon dioxide. Worse upon awakening, it subsides shortly after. Headaches may also follow long afternoon naps.

10. **CHANGES IN PERSONALITY.** Poor sleep consolidation and daytime sleepiness can produce personality changes and abnormal behavioral outbursts.

WEIGHT LOSS *with* DIET EXERCISE STRESS REDUCTION

11. SEXUAL DYSFUNCTION. Decreased sexual drive and reports of impotence have been reported.

12. HEARING LOSS. Mild hearing loss has been reported with heavy snoring during the night, especially with high decibel levels.

If you suspect you or your sleep partner is suffering from sleep apnea, I encourage you to visit your primary physician for the proper referral and testing.

We are more concerned with allowing natural sleep to occur. For the present discussion, we will assume there are no significant sleep conditions or illnesses that cannot be alleviated by following the DES principles.

75. Good quality sleep is essential for normal body and mind functioning.

CIRCADIAN RHYTHM AND SLEEP

We usually refer to the circadian rhythm as the internal clock that regulates the timing between sleep and wakefulness during the 24-hour day-night cycle. Many bodily functions occur during this 24-hour timeframe, including hormonal secretions, body temperature regulation, sensory processing, and memory performance. These daily rhythms are generated by an internal, self-sustaining, clock-like mechanism. Circadian means "about the day" and is used to describe these 24-hour day-night changes. The circadian rhythm can be affected by photic stimulation: light. This helps train the circadian rhythm to the day-night environment. Light can shift our sleep patterns. Light pushes the sleep cycle. If exposure is in the morning, it will push earlier (awaken earlier). If light exposure is in the evening, it pushes the sleep cycle to later in the night (you will want to stay awake longer). Adding to this phenomenon is the fact that the circadian rhythm is coupled to an internal clock that is not of 24-hour duration. The exact duration of a day on the planet Earth (time to complete one full spin on its axis) is 23 hours and 56 minutes. On the planet Mars, it is 24 hours and 37 minutes. Internal free-running rhythms (without a clock or imposed 24-hour light-dark period) will vary among species, ranging from 23 hours to 26 hours. In humans, it is closer to 25 hours than to 24 hours. It is actually closer to the Martian day than to Earth's! This is, of course, irrelevant to the discussion of the circadian rhythm but serves as fodder for conspiracy theories.

76. Exposure to light can affect sleep patterns dramatically.

If light can exert such a powerful influence on the quality and timing of sleep, then we must be respectful of its power. Our internal clock, and thus bedtimes, can be affected by exposure to light. Too much light and we shift the clock to later and later bedtimes. This can be a problem for school-age children and adults who have scheduled work times. This is known as delayed sleep phase syndrome. If we awaken and are exposed to light, it will also shift the internal clock to earlier times. Unfortunately, shifts occur in small increments, anywhere between 5 to 15 minutes. So, it would be difficult to correct a three-hour shift when we can only move about 10 minutes a day. As we get older, it is much more difficult to manipulate the sleep-wake schedule. It is best to be aware that this bedtime shifting can occur and attempt to catch it early by establishing and keeping good sleep schedules. School-age children during summer breaks will go to sleep later and later each night until parents realize that they are up until the wee hours of the morning. The children then want to awaken at noon as the sleep cycle has shifted. Once school starts, they are forced to wake up early, until they adjust to the new schedule once again. They can adjust fairly rapidly, and by the end of the first or second week, they are back to the school schedule. As you get older, this becomes more difficult to correct.

77. Excessive use of tablets and smartphones can disrupt sleep and cause delayed sleep phase.

We may not be aware of some of the negative aspects of screen media time (smart phones, tablets, TV). There is an association between screen-based activities and academic performance in children and adolescents. The more screen time the worse the academic performance. Screen-based activities usually occur in the evenings and night and can play a role in sleep deprivation and poor-quality sleep which has been shown to cause poor academic performance. Teenagers are more prone to have these problems because of gaming, social media, and increased screen time with light exposure to the phone.

How do you know if your clock has shifted? Just make a note of the times you awaken on the days you have not set an alarm, such as weekends. If you awaken spontaneously around the same time, give, or take 30 minutes, you have not shifted and are most likely are getting enough sleep throughout the week. That is why we emphasize setting and keeping regular sleep schedules, even on weekends or days off. If you have delayed sleep phase, your brain will not be fully awake and alert until the afternoon, since the first part of the morning, the brain is still functionally asleep. Children will do poorly with the morning classes but do quite well in the afternoon when the brain is more alert. The same goes for college students. Adults may have a difficult time getting their day started and are less productive in the mornings. Some people are "wired" with the shifted sleep cycle (genetic). These people are "night owls" and work best in the evenings and night. They have delayed sleep phase syndrome and cannot adjust to daytime jobs. Your neighborhood bartender is probably one of them.

THE GLYMPHATIC SYSTEM

78. Sleep helps rid the brain of toxins.

Sleep also plays a role in detoxifying the central nervous system (CNS). You are constantly being exposed to numerous toxins that take a toll on the immune system, liver, as well as other body mechanisms used to detoxify the brain. Sleep is one of the methods the brain uses to clear itself of toxins. These toxins can include pesticides, neurotoxins, herbicides, byproducts of metabolism, and even artificial sweeteners, which are also considered toxins. These may bind with certain receptors and potentially cause the death of a neuron. The process by which sleep helps detoxify the brain is unique. As we sleep, the cerebrospinal fluid enters the brain tissue as neurons shrink. As they shrink, the fluid surrounds the cells and in-between spaces and washes the toxins from the brain including beta amyloid which is accumulated in the brains of people with Alzheimer's. Upon awakening, the cells return to normal size, and the fluid is drained, ridding the brain of the toxins. This process is now known as the glymphatic system. The glymphatic system is a recently discovered lymphatic and detoxifying system of the brain described by Dr. Maiken Nedergaard.

 WEIGHT LOSS *with* DIET EXERCISE STRESS REDUCTION

SLEEP HYGIENE

79. Follow good sleep hygiene principles to obtain good quality sleep.

There are instructions on how to sleep! Do not throw away the instructions or consider them only when things go wrong. Good sleepers do not necessarily follow sleep hygiene principles as they sleep well and are not affected the same way as, say insomniacs. But if you are having problems sleeping, it would help to develop good sleep hygiene habits.

1. Go to sleep only when you are sleepy.
2. Keep regular sleep hours.
3. Limit caffeine consumption in the evenings. Caffeine has a half-life of 2-7 hours in young people. With increasing age, this increases to as much as 10 hours in some older people. Even low doses of caffeine consumed earlier in the day can affect sleep.
4. Avoid catch-up sleep on weekends as it has been shown to be inferior to sleeping in a more regular day-to-day schedule.
5. Avoid alcohol 3 to 4 hours prior to sleep.
6. Avoid exercise three hours prior to sleep.
7. Avoid watching TV in bed; use the bed only for sleep and sex.
8. Avoid daytime naps. Napping improves your levels of alertness but reduces your drive to sleep at night. Napping at different times during the day and of different durations can certainly disrupt sleep.
9. Avoid anxiety and stress-inducing activities prior to sleep.
10. Avoid smoking one hour prior to sleep.
11. Avoid eating nighttime snacks that increase stomach acid.
12. Avoid large amounts of liquids in the evening, thus reducing disrupted sleep from bathroom trips.
13. Do not fall asleep with the TV on. Incorporate turning off the TV as part of your sleep ritual.
14. Optimize your sleep environment, such as temperature, noise, and light level. This would include your phone.

DES CONCEPTS STEP THREE

DIET

You have already participated in the DES cleansing diet, lifetime diet and have begun an exercise program as well as stress reduction techniques. Is it enough? As you have been reading, you may ask yourself why are there so many favorable associations with the vegetarian diet? Most people believe they cannot sustain such a diet. I would recommend a slow transition to one of the four previously mentioned dietary groups. This would include the **semivegetarians**, the **pescovegetarians** (fish is ok), the **lactoovovegetarians** (milk and eggs are ok), and the vegans and strict **vegetarians**. Reduction in the incidence of diabetes, hypertension, and weight occurs with each subsequent diet. We have already discussed the fact that the microbiota and our palates will change as we adapt to these diets. I would certainly start by reducing the total amount of animal protein consumed, including poultry.

So far, you have eliminated sodas, fruit juices, seed oils, desserts, inflammatory foods, and ultra-processed foods. You have been very careful not to overindulge on potatoes, and you have been splurging on vegetables. The dietary balancing act between maintaining normal sugars and reasonable weight is compromised further by reducing cholesterol and saturated fats in the diet. DES Step Three is a voluntary dietary transition to less animal meat. I call this the half-fish diet. You do not necessarily eat half a fish, but rather, you eat fish half the time. This could include canned fish, shrimp, lobster, crab, and other shellfish. You can start this step when you are ready and have adjusted to your new pantry foods. You again follow the DES principles and attempt to eat only twice a day, a brunch around 11:30 in the morning and dinner around 6 to 7 PM. Snack in the evening if you need to and make it nuts, chocolate (1 ounce or less), avocado, or cheese (small portions such as an ounce or ounce and a half). Fruit would be acceptable, but not with a high glycemic index and preferably a berry. Now for the difficult part. You will need to reduce the amount of animal meat you eat. Strive for a 33% reduction at first. It can be easy; no meat every third meal. If you have two meat meals in a row, then the next one should be meat-free. You can also eat fish instead of meat. When eating meat, portions should be reduced to four or five ounces. Make them lean cuts, grass-fed, skinless, and trim the fat. As it becomes easier to follow, you can increase the meat-free meals to half the time. That would reduce your poultry and red meat consumption by 50%, and you have learned that substituting an egg, tofu and meat substitutes for fish will also achieve the same goal of reducing total meat consumption. See the sample recipes at the end of the book.

   WEIGHT LOSS *with* DIET EXERCISE STRESS REDUCTION

80. Reducing the amount of animal protein can decrease the incidence of diabetes, weight gain, and hypertension.

81. When it comes to the risk of cardiovascular disease, poultry is just as harmful as red meat.

The common belief is that poultry is a safe alternative to beef. Unfortunately, this is not true. Yes, it is less detrimental without the skin and cleaning the fat, However, studies have shown that poultry, white meat, and red meat are all the same when it comes to atherosclerotic heart disease (hardening of the coronary arteries). Even fish can increase the risks, but less so.

During the cleanup, it was difficult to rid yourself of the desire to consume more carbohydrates and sweets. As time went by, however, it became easier. Then it was easy to the point where you did not want to have anything too sweet. The way you make this transition is to become a semivegetarian and consume meat only 66% of the time. If this is not too difficult then try to reduce consumption to 50% or even 33% of the time, and the result is a diet you can live with. The best way to accomplish this is to have a plant protein and a base grain you can fall back on. My fallback protein is beans. We are now substituting animal protein with plant protein. A list of the protein content of several foods, including fish, is contained in Appendix-F. Remember that pescovegetarians (fish eaters) have a 50% decrease in the incidence of diabetes. The glycemic index for most beans averages around 20 to 30. The glycemic load for 150 g (a third of a cup or 5 ¼ oz) is less than 10.

82. Basmati rice, pasta, yams, green bananas, tubers, and root vegetables are all good substitutes for high glycemic index (GI) carbohydrates.

You then need to select a base grain you can fall back on. I did say grain, which means carbohydrate. My fallback grain is basmati rice. For basmati rice the glycemic index (GI) is in the low 50s and glycemic load less than

20. If you select a grain or starch, it must have a low glycemic index (less than 55). Potatoes are notoriously poor choice. Yams have a glycemic index of 54 and could be a possible substitute. Not to be confused with sweet potato, yams are a food staple of Africa and are a root vegetable and that is usually starchier and drier than sweet potato. There are over 600 varieties of yams, and they are most difficult to find in grocery stores. Sweet potato has a glycemic index of 70 which makes for a poor substitute. Pasta could be a good substitute if you watch the quantity (load). It is boiled in water that is later discarded which reduces the glycemic index. Another bit of information about basmati rice is that it is not all the same. It appears that basmati rice with high amylase content have the lowest GI scores. This basmati rice tends to be less sticky and cooks firmer. Basmati rice varieties that come from Sri Lanka seem to be the best for this. Another trick to reduce the GI of rice is to wash the rice before cooking. Then finally, there is a cooking technique in which the amount of water you first use is irrelevant. You wait until the rice is cooked to your liking and then drain and cover it.

Poor nutrition, deconditioning, and overindulgence of certain types of foods are the main reasons we gain weight, and have shortened life expectancies, hypertension, diabetes, gastrointestinal complaints, memory problems, joint pain, muscle pain, etc.

High cholesterol can be a problem. It can be part of the metabolic syndrome (to be discussed later,) inherited or due to poor dietary habits.

Some DES concepts seem to be repetitive, but in a sense, they are too important not to repeat.

80. Reducing the amount of animal protein in the diet can decrease the incidence of diabetes, weight gain, heart disease, and hypertension.

81. When it comes to the risk of cardiovascular disease, poultry is just as harmful as red meat.

82. Basmati rice, pasta, yams, green bananas, tubers, and root vegetables are all good substitutes for high glycemic index carbohydrates.

The final DES concepts relate to medical conditions, chemicals that are in your diet and metabolic syndrome.

83. Migraine headaches may respond favorably to avoiding certain headache producing foods.

84. A leaky gut, dysfunctional microbiota, and the resultant nutrient deficiency can cause restless legs syndrome.

85. Most people with non-celiac gluten sensitivity go undiagnosed and untreated. They may present without gastrointestinal symptoms and, at times, only with neurological symptoms.

86. Celiac disease and non-celiac gluten sensitivity can initiate inflammatory processes that can produce and perpetuate autoimmune diseases.

87. The current testing protocols for non-celiac gluten sensitivity are unreliable. Only 24% of those with partial villous atrophy actually test positive.

88. Lectins may make certain individuals ill; in which case they should be eliminated from the diet.

89. Phytic acid may interfere with the absorption of zinc, iron, and calcium. It may contribute to these mineral deficiencies over time.

90. Some individuals have a difficult time with fermentable sugars and may need to eliminate these offending foods. (FODMAPs)

91. It is thought that fibromyalgia may be an autoimmune disease and mediated through a leaky gut.

92. Certain foods and dysfunctional microbiota can produce goitrogenic (goiter producing) chemicals.

93. People with thyroid disease need to avoid goitrogenic foods or at least limit the amount consumed.

94. Type II diabetes and Alzheimer's disease share common enzymatic pathways that could lead to the accumulation of amyloid beta.

95. One of the first stages in the development of Type II diabetes is metabolic syndrome.

THE DES CONCEPTS BY TARGET ORGANS

BRAIN

IMPROVEMENT OF MEMORY

No one goes to sleep with perfect memories and awakens the next day with Alzheimer's disease. There is a zone, if you will, that separates normalcy from dementia. This zone is known as MCI or mild cognitive impairment. MCI is at the forefront of dementia research as it appears that 25% of people over the age of 65 have MCI. Of these, only one in three will progress and develop Alzheimer's disease. Medical science has been trying to identify what markers or environmental aspects distinguish MCI from Alzheimer's disease. How can we anticipate or predict who will progress and who will remain with MCI? Currently, we have no clear answers to these questions. We perform repeated testing and those with neurodegenerative diseases such as Alzheimer's disease, will have worsening scores as years go by. People that remain with MCI show no significant degree of progression. We have made some progress, as we know that certain activities will slow down the progression of Alzheimer's disease. These individuals adapt certain aspects of the DES concepts and improve or stop progression. But if they do have the disease, there will be eventual progression. In my experience, progressing through this zone is inevitable; thus, the people with MCI who have Alzheimer's disease will eventually worsen and, with time, begin to demonstrate signs of the disease. We were performing memory testing every six months. Usually, for the first six months after adapting some of the DES concepts, the scores improved. The following six months the scores appear unchanged, although this has been somewhat variable. When we repeat the testing a year and a half to two years out, we begin to see the progression through the MCI zone. By following the DES concepts, these people have bought themselves one or two good years of functionality and ability to perform activities of daily living with a disease that is progressive and relentless.

The following are supplements and recommendations by the Academy of Neurology for the improvement of memory.

  WEIGHT LOSS *with* DIET EXERCISE STRESS REDUCTION

1. **OMEGA-3 SUPPLEMENTS**: The Academy of Neurology recommends taking omega-3 supplements especially if it is high in DHA. At one time it was recommended we use ginkgo biloba; however, there were discrepancies in dosing between brands as there are no clear regulations in the manufacture of these supplements. Ginkgo biloba is no longer recommended for this reason. The substitute supplement was vitamin E; however, the doses required to achieve improvement caused an increase in cardiac events. Recent studies show that eating fish two to three times a week was even better and superior to taking omega-3 supplements.

2. **FOLIC ACID SUPPLEMENTS**: It has been shown that this supplement by itself along with vitamin B-12 did very little to change the course of the illness. However, in my experience those who have high homocysteine levels will benefit from the supplement. This can be measured in a blood test. Currently, I recommend using it only as an option.

3. **MULTIVITAMIN**: I cannot understand why there are advocates against the use of a multivitamin. The way I see it a multivitamin with minerals contains 20 to 25 vitamins and minerals. How can anybody be sure that they are not deficient in any one of these? The only way to be certain that there are no deficiencies is to take a multivitamin. Once you have been on the vitamin for a few months, if you want, discontinue taking it for a few months, but I would never advocate not taking one.

4. **ASPIRIN 81 MG**: There is considerable controversy surrounding the use of aspirin. This is also optional to a certain degree. Aspirin is recommended If you have a risk factor such as hypertension, diabetes, abnormal cholesterol, a family history of stroke or heart attack, abnormalities of your lipid panel, and so on, as long as there are no bleeding problems.

THINKING OUTSIDE THE BOX

A recent study performed by the National Institute on Aging (NIA) identified antioxidants that may help protect the brain from oxidative stress, which can cause cell damage. Individuals with the highest serum levels of lutein, zeaxanthin, and beta-cryptoxanthin were less likely to have dementia decades later than their peers with lower levels of those antioxidants. Zeaxanthin is a pigment that imparts red, orange, or yellow pigment in certain foods, such as **paprika, corn, saffron, goji berries, and spirulina.** Lutein and beta-cryptoxanthin can be found in green leafy vegetables, especially dark green vegetables such as **kale, spinach, turnip greens, collard greens, romaine lettuce, watercress, Swiss chard, and mustard greens.** These can be easily added to your diet. As far as additional supplements are concerned, the Academy of Neurology has yet to adapt other supplements that have been shown to be helpful in certain realms of cognitive functioning. For instance, **turmeric** has been shown in recent studies to improve verbal memory. **Vitamin D** has been helpful in improving executive function (planning ahead) and in verbal function. Studies that have used vitamin D were inconclusive and it was thought that Vitamin D would not to be helpful in delaying the progression of Alzheimer's disease. However, it was unclear if these individuals were vitamin D deficient. I will only add this supplement if the vitamin D levels are low. Approximately 60% or more of people have vitamin D insufficiency. It should be noted that there is such a thing as vitamin D toxicity. It is important to monitor levels.

The amino acid supplement **NAC** (n-acetylcysteine) seems to improve visual-spatial orientation dramatically. It also seems to help memory. There are a few other benefits to the use of NAC. It is a very strong antioxidant and helps detoxify the liver; it can reduce insulin-resistant syndrome, improve the immune system, and chelate (bind and eliminate) heavy metals, including lead, arsenic, and mercury. It has antiviral and anticancer properties. It helps protect the hippocampus (memory banks) from ischemia (lack of oxygen). It increases the production of glutathione, which is a very strong antioxidant that in itself is beneficial to the immune

  WEIGHT LOSS *with* DIET EXERCISE STRESS REDUCTION

system, improves insulin sensitivity, and has anticancer properties. Because NAC does chelate metals it should never be taken with your multivitamin and minerals as it will chelate iron, zinc, copper, and other beneficial metals. It should also not be taken with L-glutamine as they compete for absorption. I also found that if taken with Zicam, the OTC medicine used to lessen cold symptoms, it will shorten the duration of your cold or even abort it altogether. I recommend NAC 1200 mg with a Zicam at the onset of the first symptoms and allow 30 min between the two. You may have to repeat it 6 to 12 hours later.

There have been several programs to improve Alzheimer's disease symptoms that use the DES concepts (not by that name) and recommend exercise, meditation or prayer, a gluten-free diet, reduction of simple sugars, and following the Mediterranean diet (UCLA study). The DES program encompasses all of these and does so in more detail.

All the above recommendations can be used to improve memory for individuals who have no cognitive disease process. Taking **NAC, turmeric, Berberin, and enzyme Q10** (in those taking a statin*) once a day, preferably in the morning, can be used to improve memory. You may also want to add supplements of **brown seaweed,** as this has also been shown to be helpful in alleviating the symptoms of mild cognitive impairment by favorably modifying the microbiome. Overall, following the DES concepts can improve memory functions.

* Drugs used to lower cholesterol

AMYLOID BETA (ABETA)

You may have heard of this substance in the news and related to Alzheimer's disease. Amyloid beta is a combination of several amino acids that are believed to be involved in the cause of Alzheimer's disease. It is derived from the amyloid precursor protein (APP), which is broken down by enzymes to yield amyloid beta, sometimes called beta amyloid. This, in turn, can produce other compounds that are toxic to nerve cells.

Recent research is geared towards reducing the amount of amyloid beta in the brain in hopes of stopping or preventing the disease altogether. Beta amyloid accumulation is associated with memory decline. People that had increased physical activity were found to have less beta amyloid burden and thus less cognitive decline and grey matter loss. Weight loss diets are associated with improved cognitive function in obese individuals. Nearly half of dementia cases could be prevented or delayed. The list of risk factors includes hypertension, little or no education, hearing impairment, smoking, obesity, depression, physical inactivity, diabetes, and low social contact. More recently, additional risk factors have been added to the list of preventable cases of dementia to include head injuries, excessive alcohol consumption in midlife, and air pollution exposure in later life.

HEADACHES

We have known for a long time that there are dietary triggers to the onset of headaches. People who experience migraines have known for a long time that drinking red wine, eating chocolate, and certain other alcoholic beverages would trigger a migraine. A headache is the brain's response to an imbalance and disease. It is predominantly a chemical problem. Of course, you develop a headache if you have a tumor, infection, or systemic disease. However, this would manifest differently and could be picked up on physical examination and other tests. Assuming the individual does not have any of the previously mentioned conditions, when a headache occurs, there is an imbalance, mainly a chemical one. This is so true for migraine. The chemical changes related to the menstrual cycle contribute to triggering headache. Of course, the chemical responses to foods can also trigger a headache. Other triggers include changes in barometric pressure, flickering lights, stress, skipping meals, and use of certain medications. Appendix B has the usual suspects when it comes to diet-induced migraine triggers.

There are a few items on the list that merit mentioning, as they may be considered healthy. These would include nuts, yogurt, bananas, avocado, and citrus fruits. Doctors are always encouraging us to eat more fruit, and yogurt is used for gut health as a probiotic. Avocado is the cure-all in many diets. Nuts are considered the cornerstone of weight loss, good fiber intake, and overall gastrointestinal health. For those with migraines, these foods could pose a problem. I feel that diet changes can reduce migraine frequency to manageable levels in 60% of sufferers. Other treatments would include preventive medications, abortive agents, and, if all else fails, symptomatic treatment. You avoid the dietary triggers, prevent with a daily medication, abort with a medication you would take if only you had a migraine, and treat symptomatically by darkening the room, resting in bed, hydrating, etc.

83. Migraine headaches may respond favorably to avoiding certain headache producing foods.

You are wondering, what are the most common foods that trigger migraines? In adolescents: chips! They love the flavored ones. Unfortunately, instead of two to three ingredients, the side panel has a list in a very long paragraph. Somewhere in the middle, you have monosodium glutamate, which is a strong vasodilator and can trigger migraines, especially in children. In college-age young adults, it is pizza. It has cheese, pepperoni, and yeast, all known to produce headaches. They usually down it with a diet drink with artificial sweeteners that also triggers migraine. In middle-aged adults, it is wine, beer, and hard liquor. Chocolate is high on the list, as are the diet drinks.

RESTLESS LEGS SYNDROME

As the term implies, restless legs refer to an irresistible urge to move the legs. The diagnosis is usually made using the acronym U R G E. The "U" stands for the urge to move the legs, the "R" refers to occurring during rest, "G" refers to feeling better when the person gets up and walks around, and the "E" refers to the time of occurrence which usually is in the evenings when attempting to sleep. There are multiple causes of restless legs, including genetics. However, it is most common in certain deficiency states, such as iron deficiency or certain vitamin deficiencies. With celiac and non-celiac gluten sensitivity, there is malabsorption of nutrients, which can lead to restless legs as the only manifestation. Another spectrum of this disease is periodic limb movement disorder. The so-called nocturnal myoclonus. This is when a person kicks in his sleep. This is usually not a problem unless the person awakens or accidentally hits the sleeping partner. It can be treated similarly as restless legs.

84. A leaky gut and resultant nutrient deficiencies can cause restless legs syndrome.

OTHER NEUROLOGICAL DISEASES

Multiple sclerosis is an autoimmune disease that affects the central nervous system. Gastrointestinal microbiota is essential for the development and maturation of the immune system, and it is not surprising it is implicated in the pathogenesis of multiple sclerosis. The microbiota has been implicated in regulating myelin production in mice and maintaining blood-brain barrier integrity. There is even evidence that the administration of certain bacteria that produce short-chain fatty acids may reverse the loss of blood-brain barrier integrity.

Autism spectrum disorder is another condition in which a strong gene-environment interaction is involved. It is important to note that autism spectrum disorder is associated with a high incidence of gastrointestinal symptoms. There have been some studies showing changes in the microbiota can actually improve symptomatology in these individuals. There is ongoing research in this field.

Parkinson's disease is also implicated as possibly starting in the gut. An abnormal protein that deposits in the neurons responsible for the cause of Parkinson's (alpha- synuclein) has also been identified in the nerve fibers and ganglia in the intestines of those with Parkinson's syndrome. It is thought that the protein is transported to the brain via the vagus nerve. The relationship between gut proteins and cognitive health is receiving increased attention because bacteria can produce amyloid-like proteins. These studies are also ongoing. Neurotoxins in milk (organochlorine residues) have also been implicated in causing Parkinson's disease.

DES AND THE GASTROINTESTINAL TRACT

We have been discussing the benefits of a healthy microbiota. The gastrointestinal tract may be the target of a dysfunctional microbiome. The cause of many gastrointestinal illnesses remains obscure. Still, we do know a few scientific facts that may serve as a guide to at least control some of the symptoms:

1. Diet can impact symptom severity.
2. There is an inflammatory component to all these diseases.
3. Autoimmune processes may play a role in the cause and severity of these diseases.

The gastrointestinal tract can manifest disease in many ways: intermittent diarrhea, chronic diarrhea, intermittent constipation, chronic constipation, bloating, bloody stools, dark tarry stools, abdominal pain, etc. Specific illnesses can include ulcerative colitis, Crohn's disease, irritable bowel syndrome (IBS), and to be inclusive, the "leaky gut," the result of a dysfunctional microbiome. It is the antigens entering the bloodstream that promote the formation of antibodies against substances that normally are not in the blood but rather should remain in the gut. I believe some form of immune activation occurs when these substances go into the bloodstream. As with many vaccines, "cross talk" can occur, and part of the antigen protein sequence can mimic part of a body substance.

GLUTEN SENSITIVITY

85. Most people with non-celiac gluten sensitivity go undiagnosed and untreated. It may present without gastrointestinal symptoms and at times only with neurological symptoms.

A person without gluten enteropathy (the true Celiac disease) can become gluten sensitive. Gluten enters the bloodstream through the leaky gut; antibodies are produced against part of the protein that, in turn, cross-react with the villi in the small intestine, where gluten causes inflammation and eventually destroys it. This person may not test positive for Celiac disease but is now gluten sensitive. Depending on who you read, non-celiac gluten sensitivity has a prevalence of 20 to 40% of the population. In contrast, Celiac disease has a prevalence of less than 5%. This mechanism may also be responsible for many autoimmune diseases, as antibodies to other types of proteins produce unwanted damage to the brain, gut, joints, and muscles. Autoimmune diseases associated with gluten sensitivity can include non-Hodgkin's lymphoma, rheumatoid arthritis, asthma, inflammatory bowel disease, and certain cancers. An unhealthy microbiota can occur when the diet is high in carbohydrates and sugar, and low in fiber. It can be affected by environmental and foodborne toxins. Stress can also be a factor, be it acute or chronic. Infections and the use of certain medications such as antibiotics, nonsteroidal anti-inflammatory drugs, and proton pump inhibitors can also be unhealthy for the microbiome.

86. Celiac disease and non-celiac gluten sensitivity can initiate immunological processes that can produce and perpetuate autoimmune diseases.

Are celiac disease and non-celiac gluten sensitivity reversible? I do not know the full answer. I do believe changing the diet can reduce symptoms of rheumatoid arthritis, IBS, gastrointestinal complaints, and even improve brain fog, but can it reverse the process? I believe it can reduce the symptoms. Once you no longer have a leaky gut, the immune system will calm down and eventually "forget" those abnormal proteins. Of course, once you are re-exposed, you can reinitiate the inflammatory process. Many believe that non-celiac gluten sensitivity is never cured. One of these is Dr. Thomas O'Bryan. He advocates total gluten abstinence for both people with Celiac disease and those with non-celiac gluten sensitivity. Similarly, Dr. David Perlmutter bases his dietary advice on the same principle of gluten avoidance. Both medical experts are at the forefront of functional medicine. I share the same belief as Dr. Kellman, author of the "Microbiome diet" who believes that the gut can heal enough to tolerate small amounts of gluten. The exception being the true Celiac patient.

87. The current testing protocols for non-celiac gluten sensitivity are unreliable. Only 24% of people with partial villous atrophy actually test positive.

What other chemicals can activate the immune system?

LECTINS

One other culprit in the possible cause of a leaky gut is a protein called lectin. This protein is found in plants and is used by plants to protect themselves. Plants produce lectins to defend themselves from birds and insects. When insects and birds consume lectins, they become ill, and it is, in a sense, nature's natural insecticide. Some people will consume plants high in lectin. Most will have absolutely no symptoms; however, there is a small percentage that may become ill. Humans are unable to digest lectins, so they transit through the gut without being digested. Lectins seem to bind to glycoproteins and certain sugars. Some theories suggest that lectin induced-inflammation occurs as it binds to the gut wall. Research shows that cooking, fermenting, and sprouting foods that are high in lectins will reduce the total amount of present. Foods high in lectins include:

- → kidney beans
- → soybeans
- → tomatoes
- → wheat
- → peanuts.

Potatoes can be added to the list for some people. These foods are healthy. They are high in fiber and, for the most part, have a low glycemic index. Most of the lectins in tomatoes are concentrated in the skin and the seeds. This must have been known to the Italians a long time ago, as they incorporated removing skins and seeds from the tomatoes in preparing their sauces. The same goes for beans. Soaking and partially fermenting beans are old cooking techniques of our grandparents. The modern way would be to use a pressure cooker, which effectively eliminates the lectin load. If you think you have problems with lectins, you may want to go on an elimination diet for a while. Reduce or eliminate the five items mentioned above for a week or two including the nightshade vegetables (Appendix C).

88. Lectins may make certain individuals ill; in which case they should be eliminated from the diet.

89. Phytic acid may interfere with the absorption of zinc, iron, and calcium. It may contribute to these mineral deficiencies over time.

NIGHTSHADES

Nightshades are a large and diverse family of plants. These plants are poisonous, especially when unripe. Some of the more well-known plants in this family include ornamentals such as the Belladonna, Datura, Brugmansia (angel's trumpet), and Nicotonia (tobacco), all of which have poisonous properties and can cause anything from skin irritation, rapid heartbeat, hallucinations, seizures, and even death. Several vegetables belong to this group of plants that we eat on a regular basis. Some individuals are particularly sensitive to the chemicals in this group of plants. The most known are:

- tomato
- eggplant
- potato
- peppers

Like lectins, the nightshade family can also cause some health problems. It may cause intermittent problems with digestion, vomiting, dry mouth, and confusion. The nightshades contain chemicals that may be toxic to some people, and eliminating the nightshades may be beneficial to this group of people. Dr. Gundry is an advocate of eliminating the nightshades as they can contribute to health issues.

PHYTIC ACID

Phytic acid is a natural substance found in plant seeds. Its concern in nutrition has to do with the fact that they impair the absorption of iron, zinc, and calcium and may promote mineral deficiencies. Not all news about phytic acid is bad; it is a potent antioxidant, provides dietary phosphorus and may reduce the risk of colon cancer. It can protect against kidney stones. Even though the amount of these minerals can be reduced in high-phytate (phytic acid) foods, this is rarely of concern in those who follow well-balanced diets. Several methods can be used to reduce the phytic acid content of foods, including soaking, sprouting, and fermentation. See Appendix D for list of high-phytate foods.

FODMAPS (FOOD SENSITIVITY, IBD, GLUTEN SENSITIVITY TRIGGERS)

Fermentable oligosaccharides, disaccharides, monosaccharides, and polyols (FODMAPS) are increasingly being recognized as playing a role in producing symptoms in people with irritable bowel syndrome, chemical sensitivity, and even non-celiac gluten intolerance. Symptoms produced by these components include abdominal pain, bloating, flatus (wind), and altered bowel habits. There is evidence that certain food components can contribute to symptoms through the effect of malabsorption of carbohydrates and stimulation of hypersensitivity to food chemical ingestion. This may be important in people with irritable bowel syndrome but also in those that have food chemical sensitivity and even the possibility of inducing symptoms in non-celiac gluten intolerance. Short-chain carbohydrates would include lactose, fructose, and sorbitol. Other carbohydrates involved can include fructose oligosaccharides (fructans) and galacto-oligosaccharides (GOS), as they are also short-chain carbohydrates and are incompletely absorbed in the human gastrointestinal tract. The incompletely absorbed sugar polyols, sorbitol, and mannitol are used in artificial sweeteners. They are also found naturally in foods and can also be potential triggers. Eliminating FODMAPs has been described as a potential treatment for asthma, rhinitis, eczema, and even attention deficit disorder. Evidence for the use of the elimination of FODMAPs for the treatment of these conditions is still inconclusive. A FODMAP list can be found in Appendix E.

90. Some individuals have a difficult time with fermentable sugars and may need to eliminate the offending foods.

   WEIGHT LOSS *with* DIET EXERCISE STRESS REDUCTION

DES CONCEPTS AND THE MUSCULOSKELETAL SYSTEM

Muscle is chemically activated to contract via neuronal signals (nerves) with a neurotransmitter that contacts the muscle. There are specific receptors that act as "on" switches for the muscle when that chemical enters the receptor. This chemical is the neurotransmitter acetylcholine. The area of the muscle that comes in contact with the nerve is called the neuromuscular junction. In disease states, the nerve, the muscle, or the junction may be affected. For example, when the swine flu pandemic appeared in 2009, the vaccine created to combat the spread "cross-reacted" with the protein covering the nerve and caused the destruction of the nerve itself. The disease is called Guillian-Barre. The vaccine for H1-N1 (swine flu) was given to approximately 40 million people, with a reported death toll of 25 people in a short time before the immunization was stopped. You can also get Guillain-Barre after getting a viral illness such as the flu. It is still unclear if the deaths were from the vaccine or from the flu itself. This is an extreme example of how the immune system can attack our proteins and cause autoimmune diseases. In the case of rheumatoid arthritis, there are autoantibodies against the components of the joint. You attack your joints. It should not come as a surprise that the treatments include medication that suppresses the immune system, such as prednisone. With prednisone they are treating the results of the attack (inflammation) and, to some degree, the cause (immune mediated). Is all rheumatoid arthritis caused by a leaky gut? Of course not, but by avoiding the activation of the immune system you can reduce symptoms.

FIBROMYALGIA

91. It is thought that fibromyalgia may be an autoimmune disease and mediated through a leaky gut.

Now, we come to the leaky gut in the concept of fibromyalgia. This condition is still somewhat of a mystery and carries with it considerable controversy. Some 35 years ago, it was considered a "psychological state of mind" that affected perimenopausal middle-aged women. It was treated with antidepressants and anxiolytics (reduce anxiety or nervousness). Curiously, I noticed it was reproducible as everybody seemed to hurt in the same places. It was present in certain disease states such as hypothyroidism, cervical or lumbar disc disease, trauma, and carpal tunnel syndrome, to give a few examples. The latter condition was what convinced me that this is a true physiological condition and not a psychological one. However, an exact cause is yet to be determined. I had many individuals present with symptoms of carpal tunnel syndrome and neck pain. When we performed electrophysiological studies on them, the carpal tunnel was confirmed, but there was nothing wrong with the neck. In fact, we would conduct CT or MRI scans and they would have totally normal scans. The physical examination however, revealed myofascial trigger points (fibromyalgia) but only on the same side of the arm and neck in which the carpal tunnel was present. Not only that, but after successful treatment of the carpal tunnel syndrome, the myofascial trigger points disappeared!

In fibromyalgia, it is thought that the electrical activity and the balance of information going to and leaving the muscle is disrupted. The neuromuscular junction is the area that hurts when you press on it (trigger point). There are no sensory nerves for perception of tingling and numbness in the neuromuscular junction that is referred to a distant site. How can you cause numbness and tingling when you press a trigger point if no nerves are going there? It is very complicated. The answer seems to be a short-circuit in the nerve-muscle connection. The signals are traveling to the muscle to make it contract, a one-way signal. However, the muscle and the joint cannot over-stretch; it must have proper control of the tension, especially for fine muscle control. It must know where the arm, joint and muscle are in space. For example, you can touch your nose with your eyes closed with exact precision without looking. All these functions come from other nerve endings that go to the brain from the neuromuscular junction and, thus, the muscle. So, there is a two-way street after all. These nerves

WEIGHT LOSS *with* DIET EXERCISE STRESS REDUCTION

do not transmit numbness or tingling so there are still some unanswered questions about how pressing on the trigger point cause sensations. I believe that the short-circuit is also occurring at the spinal cord level. Press a trigger point in the webbing of the thumb and it tingles at another nerve level supplying the forearm. The spinal cord is organized by segments. A signal enters the spinal cord and does not go straight to the brain or from the brain directly to the segment supplying the muscle or skin sensation. Rather, it sends a signal to several levels or segments up or down the spinal cord. This allows the signals to get scrambled and overlap sensory levels.

The aforementioned mechanism still does not help in determining the role of the leaky gut and autoimmune processes in fibromyalgia. Is it even related to a leaky gut? I am certain it is. At least in some people changing their diets improves symptoms dramatically, while others improve very little. Is there more than one mechanism, more than one disease? There is ongoing research to answer these questions.

THYROID HEALTH

There are substances, chemicals, and some foods that can disrupt thyroid function. This usually occurs when there is an interference with the utilization of iodine. These foods and chemicals are called goitrogens. Goitrogens are compounds that interfere with the normal function of the thyroid gland. Its interference makes it more difficult for the thyroid gland to produce hormones at normal levels. Enlargement of the thyroid gland causes a goiter. A goitrogen food can induce a goiter, and certain vegetables can affect the thyroid when consumed in excess. Some of these foods are quite healthy. Flavonoids are a goitrogen and are naturally present in a wide variety of foods. This can include **red wine** and **green tea**. They are considered healthy antioxidants, but some can be converted into goitrogenic compounds by the microbiome. We again mention a dysfunctional microbiota that can cause thyroid dysfunction. The goiter occurs when thyroid hormone production is decreased, and the pituitary attempts to increase it by producing more thyroid-stimulating hormone. The thyroid compensates by growing more cells, eventually leading to enlargement and a goiter. I will provide a list of goitrogens at the end of the section.

There are several ways to reduce the amount of goitrogens in foods. Cooking is one and probably the main technique. Steaming and boiling are others. Fermentation may actually increase the goitrogens but can reduce other compounds that could cause a goiter. Maintaining a balanced and varied diet can help, and you should limit the amount of goitrogens you consume. The take-home message from this is to know that some **raw** vegetables can interfere with the absorption and utilization of iodine. This usually happens when raw vegetables are consumed and when used in smoothies. Consuming more iodine can certainly help; keep in mind that the microbiota can interfere with the proper absorption. Iodine-containing foods include seaweed, cod, shrimp, tuna, and eggs. People with thyroid conditions should keep in mind the goitrogenic foods and attempt to consume less than one serving a day of these foods. Cruciferous vegetables are mostly those involved. These vegetables are cold weather vegetables and have flowers that have four petals, so they resemble a cross.

CRUCIFEROUS VEGETABLES:

- Bok Choi
- Broccoli
- Brussels sprouts
- Cabbage
- Cauliflower
- Collard greens
- Horseradish
- Kale
- Kohlrabi
- Mustard greens
- Rapeseed (canola)
- Rutabagas
- Spinach
- Turnips

- Bamboo shoots
- Cassava
- Corn
- Lima beans
- Linseed
- Millet
- Peaches
- Peanuts
- Pears
- Pine nuts
- Strawberries
- Sweet potatoes

SOY-BASED FOODS:

- Tofu
- Tempeh
- Edamame
- Soy milk

92. Certain foods and dysfunctional microbiota can produce goitrogenic chemicals.

93. People with thyroid disease need to avoid goitrogenic foods or at least limit the amount consumed.

TYPE II DIABETES MELLITUS

The body uses insulin for glucose to enter the cells, which in turn is used for energy. When the cells become resistant to insulin, you can develop a state of insulin resistance. If glucose cannot enter the cells easily in the presence of insulin resistance, then the sugar gets stored. This results in weight gain. The process of insulin resistance is still incompletely understood.

HIGH GLYCEMIC INDEX FOODS DIGEST
QUICKLY → EMPTY STOMACH →
INCREASED GHRELIN

RESULTS IN HUNGER

RESISTANT STARCHES DIGEST SLOWLY
→FULL STOMACH →
INCREASED LEPTIN

MAKES YOU FEEL FULL

The leptin-ghrelin relationship and the presence of hunger

There is a relationship between too many carbs and sugar and developing something we call leptin resistance. Leptin (not to be confused with lectin) helps suppress appetite. This chemical is excreted when fat cells expand, such as after a meal. Another chemical that is secreted is ghrelin, and this chemical produces hunger. It is secreted when there is an empty stomach. If you eat a fast-digesting food, such as one with a high glycemic index, you will feel hunger much more frequently throughout the day. You become more resistant to leptin as you consume more sugar and carbohydrates. Weight gain undoubtedly ensues.

The same enzymes that break down insulin also break down amyloid beta. Increasing insulin reduces the brain's ability to break down amyloid beta, and this can accumulate in the brain. It is thought that this abnormal

    WEIGHT LOSS *with* DIET EXERCISE STRESS REDUCTION

protein is the cause of Alzheimer's disease and memory loss. It is no wonder that doctors sometimes call Alzheimer's disease diabetes Type III.

94. Type II diabetes and Alzheimer's disease share common enzymatic pathways that could lead to the accumulation of amyloid beta.

95. One of the first stages in the development of Type II diabetes is metabolic syndrome.

Several medical conditions occur together that will increase the risk of stroke, heart disease, and the development of Type II diabetes. These conditions are known as metabolic syndrome and include:

- Elevated blood pressure.
- High blood glucose.
- Increased cholesterol.
- Increased triglycerides.
- Increase in the amount of body fat around the waist.

The latter is the only visible sign of metabolic syndrome. The causes of metabolic syndrome include a high BMI and physical inactivity. Risk factors for metabolic syndrome include:

- Age over 45
- Ethnicity (Hispanic, African American, and Native American)
- Obesity, especially abdominal
- Increase risk of diabetes (gestational diabetes, family history of Type II diabetes)
- Nonalcoholic fatty liver (NAFL)
- Obstructive sleep apnea
- Certain medications including steroid use and antipsychotics
- Low vitamin D levels
- Polycystic ovary syndrome

Metabolic syndrome will result in a higher incidence of myocardial infarction, kidney disease, and stroke. Following the DES concepts will help prevent and treat the metabolic syndrome.

GLYCEMIC INDEX FOR COMMON FOODS

G- Contains gluten, consumption should be moderate or avoided

GI should be as close to 55 or less, >55 is in italics

FOOD	GLYCEMIC INDEX	SERVING SIZE (GRAMS)	GLYCEMIC LOAD
BAKERY PRODUCTS AND BREAD			
G- Banana cake without sugar	47	60	14
G- Banana cake with sugar	55	60	12
G- Sponge cake	46	60	17
G- Course barley bread	34	30	7
G- *Pumpernickel bread*	*56*	30	7
G- *50% cracked wheat Bread*	*58*	30	12
G- 100% Whole Grain Bread* ™	51	30	7
Corn tortilla	52	50	12
G- Wheat tortilla	30	50	8
BEVERAGES			
Apple juice, unsweetened	44	125 ml	15
Orange juice, unsweetened	50	250 ml	12
Pomegranate juice	53	200 ml	18
Tomato juice	38	250 ml	4

FOOD	GLYCEMIC INDEX	SERVING SIZE (GRAMS)	GLYCEMIC LOAD
G-Al-Bran TM	55	30	12
Oatmeal	55	250	13
G-*Special-K* TM	59	30	14
G- Pearled Barley	28	150	12
Quinoa	53	150	13
*White Basmati***	57	150	19
Brown rice	50	150	16
Converted rice, Uncle Ben's TM	38	150	14
G- Whole wheat kernels	30	50	11
G- Bulgur	48	150	12

*Brand name made by Natural Ovens

**Avoid instant and precooked as they have a higher glycemic index

60 grams=2.11 oz   150 grams=5.29 oz

FOOD	GLYCEMIC INDEX	SERVING SIZE (GRAMS)	GLYCEMIC LOAD
DAIRY PRODUCTS			
Ice cream, regular ***	57	50	6
Ice cream, premium	38	50	3
Milk, whole	41	250 ml	5
Milk, skim	32	250 ml	4
Reduced fat yogurt with fruit	33	200	11
FRUIT			
Apple	39	120	6
Apricot	34	120	4
Blueberries	25	120	2
Cherries	25	120	4
Cherry Plum	25	120	1
Grapefruit	25	120	3
Orange	40	120	4
Peach	42	120	5
Pear	38	120	4
Pomegranate	35	120	7
Prunes, pitted	29	60	10
Raspberries	25	120	3

High GI and/or GL fruit: ripe bananas, melon, canned fruit with added sugar, fig, dried apricots, mango, dried apples and dates, papaya, raisins, grapes, watermelon.

***may contain wheat (gluten) as a thickener

FOOD	GLYCEMIC INDEX	SERVING SIZE (GRAMS)	GLYCEMIC LOAD
BEANS AND NUTS			
Blackeye peas	33	150	10
Black beans	30	150	7
Chickpeas	10	150	3
Navy beans	31	150	9
Kidney beans	29	150	7
Lentils	29	150	5
Soybeans	15	150	1
Almonds	15	50	2
Cashews	27	50	3
Coconut	45	50	1
Peanuts	7	50	1
Pistachios	15	50	4
Walnuts	15	50	2

FOOD	GLYCEMIC INDEX	SERVING SIZE (GRAMS)	GLYCEMIC LOAD
PASTA AND NOODLES			
G- Fettuccini	32	180	15
G- Spaghetti	42	180	17
Mung bean noodles	25	180	19

In general pasta has a low glycemic index including gluten free pasta. Unfortunately, the glycemic load is high. You must reduce the portions in order to benefit from the low GI.

FOOD	GLYCEMIC INDEX	SERVING SIZE (GRAMS)	GLYCEMIC LOAD
SNACK FOODS			
Corn chips	42	50	11
Dark chocolate	23	100	41
Milk chocolate	50	100	41
M&M's peanut	33	30	6
Microwave Popcorn	55	20	6
Potato chips	51	50	12
Snickers bar ™	51	60	18

FOOD	GLYCEMIC INDEX	SERVING SIZE (GRAMS)	GLYCEMIC LOAD
VEGETABLES			
Green Peas	51	80	4
Carrots	35	80	2
Corn	35	100	2
Parsnips	52	80	4
Potato (instant, white boiled)	*85*	150	22
Baked russet potato	*111*	150	33
Sweet Potato	*70*	150	22
Yam	54	150	20
OTHER			
Hummus	6	30	1
G- Chicken nuggets reheated	46	100	7

A more extensive list may be obtained on the internet. A good start is the University of Sydney's site: glycemicindex.com.

100 grams=3.53 oz   180 grams=6.35 oz

SUMMARY OF THE DES CONCEPTS.

1. Diet changes can alter the microbiome.

2. Add prebiotics and probiotics during the DES cleanup diet.

3. Low carbohydrate diets outperform low-fat diets.

4. Eliminate all inflammatory foods.

5. Eliminate refined carbohydrates from the diet, or at least cut them to a minimum.

6. Sweeten only with monk fruit, Allulose, or Stevia.

7. Eliminate all desserts.

8. Never drink a soda again, be it regular or diet.

9. Avoid GMO foods when possible.

10. Reducing the consumption of animal protein and fats can result in lower incidence of heart disease and stroke.

11. The best cooking oils based on all factors are avocado and olive oils.

12. Avoid excessive use of seed oils as they can promote inflammation.

13. Eliminate all ultra-processed foods.

14. The Mediterranean diet can be as useful as the DES lifetime diet and can be followed after the cleanup diet.

15. High-protein diets increase basic metabolic rate. This higher rate is temporary and will revert to normal as the protein load diminishes.

16. Start with the DES cleanup diet as it makes it easier to follow.

17. The DES cleanup diet is a modified Paleo diet.

18. Vegetarians live longer when they follow DES principles.

19. A glass or two of red wine a day may offer invaluable benefits to your health.

20. The use of unsaturated fats, such as olive oil, can reduce the negative effects of the saturated fats in meat.

21. The use of red wine can reduce the negative impact of saturated fats in the diet.

22. You need to change your eating habits as you age.

23. Adjust your diet as you enter a new stage in life.

24. High carbohydrate and calorie-dense diets are never acceptable at any age

25. Introduce healthy carbohydrates slowly into the DES cleanup diet preferably high fiber and with a low glycemic index.

26. White sugar and high fructose corn syrup have an unacceptable glycemic index of over 70 and can lead to inflammation.

27. Genetics is only part of the picture. You need to follow healthy lifestyles (DES) in order to maximize longevity.

28. Consuming resistant starches may help with weight loss and fat burning.

29. Maximum benefits of exercise are best achieved when exercising in the mornings.

30. Partial and intermittent fasting (16-24 hours) may help in weight reduction and can be integrated into the DES diet.

31. If you want to eat breakfast, do so after exercise and make it the equal number of calories you just burned.

32. Reduce or eliminate gluten-containing foods. Even if you do not have celiac disease, refined wheat is an inflammatory food and should be consumed in small amounts.

33. Taking supplements is optional; however, many factors alter and affect proper nutrition, and supplements can help offset these factors.

34. There are supplements that help support a healthy microbiota, reduce anxiety, and help sleep.

35. There are supplements that help with hot flashes, bone loss, and diabetes.

36. There is no single supplement that will cause weight loss.

37. Some supplements help joint pain, others can help stimulate your natural growth hormone levels, and some that may help improve memory.

38. Many supplements may be detrimental to your health, especially when overdosing.

39. People with rheumatoid arthritis should be particularly careful with certain supplements which could actually cause more problems and worsen the disease.

40. The Western diet is deficient in fiber, and most people fail to consume the daily dietary minimum.

41. Try to balance the carbohydrate intake to 25-30% of your total food consumption.

42. There are fiber supplements available but increase the use of these supplements gradually to avoid side effects.

43. Avoid large portions of the sweeter fruit.

44. The Dirty Dozen list represents foods that are high in pesticide and pesticide residues.

45. Wash, scrub, and rinse your fruit and vegetables before consumption.

46. Buy organic foods and vegetables if possible.

47. Good hydration is important but try not to overdo it to avoid water intoxication.

48. Depending on your activity level, consume 4 to 8 eight-ounce glasses of water daily.

49. Filtered water is preferable to tap water. Plastic water bottles should not be allowed to be exposed to high heat.

50. You obtain roughly half of your daily water requirements from the food you eat.

51. We need to maintain muscle tone and mass by using them.

52. Get medical clearance before you start vigorous exercise programs and start slow.

53. Get some daily physical activity, even if it is just for 10 to 15 minutes.

54. Any amount of exercise is beneficial; cardio exercise is even better.

55. Three hours of aerobic exercise a week increases life expectancy by approximately ten years.

56. Walking will burn 314 cal. An hour.

57. Running more than 20 miles a week begins to undo the cardiovascular benefits of running.

58. Do not be afraid to sweat.

59. A sports watch may be helpful to keep track of your heart rate so that your pulse will remain at no more than 80% of the maximum for your age when first starting an exercise program.

60. Some sport watches can help count steps, monitor your sleep, and even tell you the recovery time needed after you work out.

61. Running shoes need to be replaced at around 300-350 miles as they tend to lose their resiliency.

62. Aerobic exercise can lower cholesterol, raise HDL, help with weight maintenance, and decrease anxiety and depression.

63. It is important to maintain an exercise regimen not just for a few weeks, but for the rest of your life.

64. Although it is not for everyone, going to the gym can motivate you to exercise.

65. There are other ways of toning muscle other than weightlifting.

66. Resistance exercises have many advantages that can help you maintain body weight and muscle tone and save time, especially with our busy schedules.

67. Stress can harm the body and mind. It can be the harbinger of disease.

68. We need to identify the sources of stress in our lives in order to deal with them and eventually reduce the negative effects they could have on our lives.

69. Biofeedback can be a tool in reducing stress.

70. Do not underestimate the power of prayer in reducing stress and helping us cope with stressful situations.

71. Tai chi and yoga are helpful in reducing stress and keeping us fit.

72. Mindfulness techniques can provide health benefits.

73. Breathing exercises can help reduce stress and are easy to do.

74. Sleep apnea can cause daytime sleepiness, fatigue, memory problems, depression, and decreased libido and can be treated with weight loss.

75. Good quality sleep is essential for normal body and mind functioning.

76. Exposure to light can affect sleep patterns dramatically.

77. Excessive use of tablets and smartphones can disrupt sleep and cause delayed sleep phase.

78. Sleep helps rid the brain of toxins.

79. Follow good sleep hygiene principles to obtain good quality sleep.

80. Reducing the amount of animal protein can decrease the incidence of diabetes, weight gain, and hypertension.

81. When it comes to the risk of heart disease, poultry is just as harmful as red meat.

82. Basmati rice, pasta, yams, green bananas, tubers, and root vegetables are all good substitutes for high glycemic index grains.

83. Migraine headaches may respond favorably to avoiding certain headache producing foods.

84. A leaky gut, dysfunctional microbiome and the resultant nutrient deficiency can cause restless legs syndrome.

85. Most people with non-celiac gluten sensitivity go undiagnosed and untreated. They may present without gastrointestinal symptoms, and at times, only with neurological symptoms.

86. Celiac disease and non-celiac gluten sensitivity can initiate inflammatory processes that can produce and perpetuate autoimmune diseases.

87. The current testing protocols for non-celiac gluten sensitivity are unreliable. Only 24% of individuals with partial villous atrophy actually test positive.

88. Lectins may make certain individuals ill; in which case they should be eliminated from the diet.

89. Phytic acid may interfere with the absorption of zinc, iron, and calcium. It may contribute to these mineral deficiencies over time.

90. Some individuals have a difficult time with fermentable sugars and may need to eliminate the offending foods. (FODMAPs)

91. It is thought that fibromyalgia may be an autoimmune disease and mediated through a leaky gut.

92. Certain Foods and a dysfunctional microbiome can produce goitrogenic chemicals.

93. People with Thyroid Disease need to avoid goitrogenic foods or at least limit the amount consumed.

94. Type II diabetes and Alzheimer's disease share common enzymatic pathways that could lead to the accumulation of amyloid beta.

95. One of the first stages in the development of diabetes Type II is metabolic syndrome.

APPENDIX A

ROOT VEGETABLES

- Beets
- Carrots
- Turnips
- Daikon
- Jerusalem artichoke
- Sweet potato
- Cassava
- Celery root
- Parsnips
- Taro root
- Potato

ROOT VEGETABLES BY GLYCEMIC INDEX (LOW TO HIGH)

LOW GI TO MODERATE GI		
Carrots	16*	
Daikon	32*	
Radish	32*	
Jerusalem Artichoke	32*	
Celery root (celeriac)	35*	*these are allowed during Step Two and Three
Cassava (yucca)	46*	
Parsnips	52*	
Taro root	54*	

BORDERLINE HIGH GI (USE SPARINGLY)	
➔ Beets	64
➔ Sweet potato	70
HIGH GI (AVOID THESE)	
➔ Turnips	73
➔ Russet Potatoes	76
➔ Boiled white Potatoes	82
➔ Mashed Potatoes	85
➔ Instant Mashed Potatoes	88
➔ Boiled Red Potatoes	89

APPENDIX B

HEADACHE TRIGGERS:

- fatigue
- sunlight
- glare
- stress
- oversleeping
- hormonal changes (menses, ovulation, birth control pills)
- environmental changes (noise, wind, smoke)
- altitude

FOODS THAT MAY TRIGGER MIGRAINE:

BEVERAGES	MEAT AND FISH	VEGETABLES
Alcohol	Aged canned/cured	Broad Beans
Buttermilk	Bologna	Fava Beans
Caffeine	Chicken livers	Lima Beans
Chocolate milk	Frankfurters	Navy Beans
BAKED GOODS	**MEAT AND FISH (CONT.)**	**VEGETABLES(CONT.)**
Fresh-Baked Breads	Marinated Meats	Onions
Sourdough Bread	Pepperoni	Peas
	Pickled Herring	Sauerkraut
	Salami	
	Sausage	

FRUITS	DAIRY	OTHER
Avocados	Aged, Processed Cheese	Chocolate
Bananas	Sour Cream	Frozen Dinners
Canned Soup	Yogurt	Garlic
Canned figs		Meat tenderizer
Citrus fruits		MSG
Papayas		Seasoned Salt
Passionfruit		Soy Sauce
Raisins		Yeast Extracts
Red Plums		Nutra-Sweet

APPENDIX C

SPECIAL ELIMINATION DIET FOR HIGH LECTIN CONTAINING FOODS

THIS COLUMN CONTAINS FOODS YOU CAN EAT FOR THE TRIAL PERIOD OF ONE OR TWO WEEKS	THIS COLUMN IS HIGH LECTIN FOODS THAT YOU WANT TO EXCLUDE DURING TRIAL PERIOD
OILS	
Avocado	Canola, soy
Coconut	Cottonseed
Olive	Corn
Sesame	Sunflower
	Vegetable Oil
	Peanut, Safflower
NUTS AND SEEDS	
Coconut Milk, Walnuts	Cashews, Sesame
Macadamia, Chestnut	Chia, Pine Nuts
Pecan, Pistachios	Peanuts, Almonds
	Pumpkin, Hazelnuts, Sunflower

THIS COLUMN CONTAINS FOODS YOU CAN EAT FOR THE TRIAL PERIOD OF ONE OR TWO WEEKS	THIS COLUMN IS HIGH LECTIN FOODS THAT YOU WANT TO EXCLUDE DURING TRIAL PERIOD
GRAINS	
Cassava, Millet, White Rice	Barley, Corn, Cornstarch
Green Bananas	Oats, Popcorn, Quinoa
Green Plantains	Brown and Wild Rice
Sesame	Rye, Spelt
Sorghum, Taro, Turnips	Wheat
Yams and Sweet Potatoes	
Yucca (most of these are grain substitutes)	
VEGETABLES	
All you can eat except those in the excluded list	Beans (and Sprouts)
	Chickpeas, Edamame
	Tofu, Hummus, Soy
	Lentils, Peas, Green Beans

THIS COLUMN CONTAINS FOODS YOU CAN EAT FOR THE TRIAL PERIOD OF ONE OR TWO WEEKS	THIS COLUMN IS HIGH LECTIN FOODS THAT YOU WANT TO EXCLUDE DURING TRIAL PERIOD
FRUIT	
Avocado, Apple, Berries	**Bell Peppers**
Dates, Kiwi, Peaches	**Chili Peppers, Eggplant**
Pears, Plums	**Cucumbers, Goji Berries**
Pomegranates	Melons, Pumpkins
	Tomatoes, Zucchini
OTHER	
Vinegars, Miso, Olives	limit Alcohol to less than two ounces daily
all spices except **Chili Pepper Flakes**	**Potatoes, Tomatillo**

The nightshade plants are in **bold**.

APPENDIX D

HIGH PHYTATE CONTAINING FOODS

GRAINS:

- → Wheat Bran
- → Rice Bran
- → Whole Wheat
- → Corn
- → Rye
- → Oats
- → Brown rice

BEANS AND NUTS:

- → Soy
- → Pinto Beans
- → Kidney Beans
- → Navy Beans
- → White Beans
- → Peas
- → Lentils
- → Chickpeas
- → Walnuts
- → Mung Beans
- → Peanuts

POTATOES:

The phytate in potatoes is not eliminated with cooking.

APPENDIX E

FODMAPs ELIMINATION DIET

FOR CHEMICALS:

1. Salicylates (can be found in fruits, vegetables, herbs, spices, nuts, tea, coffee).

2. Amines (chocolate, smoked fish, sauces, stocks, nuts, seeds, vinegar and some fruit and vegetables)

3. Monosodium Glutamate (MSG: found in strong cheeses, soy sauce and as flavor enhancer).

FOR PRESERVATIVES:

1. Benzoates
2. Propionate
3. Sulfites
4. Nitrites
5. Sorbic acid

FOR COMMON FOOD ALLERGENS:

1. Wheat
2. Dairy
3. Soy
4. Fish
5. Seafood
6. Nuts
7. Peas
8. Beans

FOR CARBOHYDRATES:

1. Sorbitol

2. Mannitol

Not all FODMAPs will be symptom triggers in all people. Only those that are malabsorbed play a role. Importantly, fructans and galacto-oligosaccharides (GOS) are always malabsorbed and fermented by intestinal microflora. This results in gas production and associated flatulence in healthy people. They may make IBS worse.

Fructans include agave, artichokes, asparagus, leaks, garlic, onions, yacon (a tuberous root), jicama and wheat.

GOS includes milk (lactose), soybean whey, sugar beet.

APPENDIX F

HIGH DIETARY PROTEIN SOURCES

MEAT GROUP:

- → Porkchops — 25 g in a 3-ounce serving
- → Chicken — 25 g in a 3-ounce serving
- → Red beef — 20 g in a 3-ounce serving (grass fed)
- → Tuna — 25 g in a 3-ounce serving
- → Salmon — 23 g in a 3-ounce serving
- → Anchovies — 20 g in a 3-ounce serving

DAIRY GROUP:

- → Buffalo mozzarella — 22 g in a 3-ounce serving
- → Cottage cheese — 25 g in a 1 cup serving
- → Cheddar cheese — 6 g in a 1 ounce serving
- → Greek yogurt — 25 g per 1 cup serving (will depend on the brand)
- → Egg — 6 g per serving (one large egg)
- → Dairy or soy milk — 8 g in 1 cup

LEGUMES:

- → Navy beans — 20 g in a 1 cup serving
- → Quinoa — 8 g in a ¾ cup serving
- → Flaxseed — 2 g in 2 tablespoons
- → Tofu — 9 g in 3 ounce serving
- → Peas — 4 g in ½ cup
- → Edamame — 13.24 g in 1 cup

SEEDS:

- → Hemp — 4 g in 1 tablespoon
- → Chia seed — 2 g in 1 tablespoon
- → Sunflower seeds — 7 g in a quarter cup
- → Amaranth — 9 g in 1 cup

VEGETABLES:

- → Avocados — 7 g in half an avocado
- → Artichokes — 4 g 1 medium
- → Mushrooms — 2.2 g in 1 cup
- → Asparagus — 3 g in 1 cup
- → Spinach — 2.8 g in half a cup

NUTS (1 OZ SERVING):

- → Pistachios — 5.94 g
- → Walnuts — 4.3 g
- → Almonds — 6 g
- → Pumpkin seeds — 7 g

OTHER:

- → Nutritional yeast   11 g in 3 tablespoons
- → California roll   6 g in five pieces
- → Corn tortilla   3 g in an 8-inch tortilla
- → Spirulina powder   8 g in 2 tablespoons

GLOSSARY

- ⊙ **ALA** – Alpha lipoic acid is a naturally occurring compound that is essential to the body and serves functions at the cellular level and energy production.

- ⊙ **AEROBIC EXERCISE** – Physical exercise dependent on oxygen energy production (cardio).

- ⊙ **ANXIOLYTICS** – Any compound that can reduce anxiety.

- ⊙ **ASHWAGANDHA** – Is an ayurvedic herb known to reduce stress.

- ⊙ **BERBERINE** – A select European herb that assists in lowering blood sugar.

- ⊙ **BETA-AMYLOID** – Is a protein derived from precursor protein in the brain and accumulates in people with Alzheimer's disease.

- ⊙ **BLACK COHOSH** – Is a member of the Buttercup family, has many uses but is primarily used to alleviate menopausal symptoms.

- ⊙ **BMI** – Body mass index considers height and weight to establish weight guidelines.

- ⊙ **BRAIN ATROPHY** – Refers to shrinkage of the brain tissue.

- ⊙ **BRUGMANSIA** – One of several species of flowering plants in the nightshade family.

- ⊙ **BUTYRATE** – Is a four-carbon short chain fatty acid and is produced when gut bacteria break down dietary fiber.

- ⊙ **CATACHINS** – A type of phenolic compound in berries, tea, and cocoa. It is a strong antioxidant.

→ **CELIAC DISEASE** – An autoimmune disease in which there is an inflammatory response in the gut to gluten, a protein in wheat and other grains.

→ **CHRYSIN** – A flavonoid found in honey, bee propolis, passionflower, and geranium.

→ **CURCUMIN** – A polyphenol obtained from the rhizome of Curcuma Longa.

→ **CYTOKINES** – Are signaling proteins that help the body's immune and inflammatory responses to biological modulators.

→ **DATURA** – A flowering plant of the nightshade family.

→ **DELAYED SLEEP PHASE** –DSP is when the circadian clock for sleep is delayed.

→ **DEMENTIA** – conditions causing memory dysfunction.

→ **DHA** – Docosahexaenoic acid is an omega-3 fat.

→ **DYSBIOSIS** – Term used to describe a dysfunctional microbiota.

→ **FEEDBACK** – Technique used to reinforce a behavior.

→ **FLAVONOID** – Plant derived phenolic metabolites with strong antioxidant properties. They are found in fruits, vegetables, grains, roots, tea, and wine.

→ **FRUCTAN** – A polymer of fructose molecules, fructooligosaccharides.

→ **GABA** – Gamma aminobutyric acid is a neurotransmitter, predominantly inhibitory.

→ **GLUTAMATE RECEPTORS** – Receptors specific for the neurotransmitter glutamate.

→ **GHRELIN** – A hormone that triggers hunger.

→ **GLA** – Gamma-linolenic acid is an omega-6 fat.

→ **GLUTEN** – A protein found in wheat, rye, barley, spelt and farro.

- ⊙ **GLYCEMIC INDEX** – Value given to a specific food compared to glucose that has a value of 100.

- ⊙ **GLYCEMIC LOAD** – Value given to a specific food based on how much it will raise the blood sugar.

- ⊙ **GLYPHOSATE** – Chemical name for the herbicide "Roundup". Thought to cause damage to the microbiome.

- ⊙ **GMO** – Genetically modified organisms are organisms that have had alterations to their DNA not occurring normally in nature.

- ⊙ **GOITROGENIC** – Promoting a goiter.

- ⊙ **HOMOCYSTEINE** – An amino acid with the methylene ridge.

- ⊙ **HONOKIOL** – A herb extracted from the bark of the magnolia tree that has a neuroprotective property and helps relaxation.

- ⊙ **HORDEINS** – A glycoprotein found in barley containing gluten.

- ⊙ **HIPPOCAMPUS** – Area of the brain involved in preserving memory.

- ⊙ **INFARCTION** – Area of tissue that lacks blood supply is dead or dying.

- ⊙ **INULIN** – A polysaccharide produced by plants, is a dietary fiber (a fructan).

- ⊙ **JICAMA** – A root vegetable in the Fabaceae family (as is peas).

- ⊙ **KETONES** – A substance used by the body when there is not enough sugar. It is formed when the body begins to burn fat for energy.

- ⊙ **KHOLRABI** – German turnip (cabbage family), can be eaten raw or cooked.

- ⊙ **LECTIN** – Carbohydrate binding proteins, can induce inflammation.

- ⊙ **LEPTIN** – A hormone made by fat cells that helps decrease hunger.

- **L GLUTAMINE** – A nonessential amino acid found in the diet. It is an energy source for the gut and helps gut health.

- **LINOLEIC ACID** – A polyunsaturated omega-6 fatty acid.

- **L-THEANINE** – An amino acid found in green tea, has calming effects.

- **MICROBIOTA** – Term used to refer to bacteria, viruses, and yeast in the gut.

- **MICROBIAL CELLS** – Alternate name applied to bacteria.

- **MICROBIOME** – Term that encompasses the entirety of the gut in relation to the human host and their interactions.

- **MELATONIN** – Hormone that helps modulate the circadian (about the day) rhythm.

- **METABOLIC SYNDROME** – A constellation of symptoms reflecting underlying chronic inflammation. These include hypertension, high cholesterol, high triglycerides, and obesity (especially around the waist).

- **METHYLSYNEPHRINE** – Artificial chemical added to supplements. It is an amphetamine and not sanctioned by the FDA (it's illegal).

- **MONOSATURATED FATS** – Have one double bonded carbon in the fatty acid chain. The rest of the carbon bonds are single bonds.

- **MUFA** – Term referring to monounsaturated fatty acids.

- **MYOCARDIAL** – In reference to the heart and myocardium.

- **NAC** – L-acetyl cysteine is a form of the amino acid cysteine.

- **NAFL** – Nonalcoholic fatty liver.

- **NEUROTOXIN** – Toxins affecting the nervous system.

- **NICOTIANA** – A plant species of wild tobacco, it's common name is tree tobacco.

- ⊙ **OMEGA-3** – Are essential polyunsaturated fatty acids characterized by the presence of a double bond, three atoms away from the terminal methyl group.

- ⊙ **OMEGA-6** – Are essential polyunsaturated fatty acids characterized by the presence of a double bond six atoms away from the terminal methyl group. Excess can cause inflammation.

- ⊙ **ORGANOCHLORINE** – Hydrocarbon-based chemical containing chlorine, used in pesticides such as DDT.

- ⊙ **PD** – Short abbreviation for Parkinson's disease.

- ⊙ **PHYTOESTROGENS** – Plant produced estrogen-like compounds.

- ⊙ **POI** – Polynesian dish made with resistant starches such as taro, breadfruit, or plantain.

- ⊙ **POLYUNSATURATED FATS** – Fats that contain two or more carbon–carbon double bonds.

- ⊙ **PREBIOTICS** – Foods that promote the growth of the beneficial bacteria in the gut.

- ⊙ **PROAMTHOCYANIDINS** – A polyphenol found in plants such as grapes, cranberry, blueberry.

- ⊙ **PROBIOTICS** – Live organisms taken orally to replenish the microbiome.

- ⊙ **PROLAMINS** – Plant protein with a high proline acid content.

- ⊙ **PROLINE** – An organic amino acid that enhances the production of proteins.

- ⊙ **PUFA** – Abbreviated form for polyunsaturated fatty acid.

- ⊙ **RESISTANT STARCHES** – A starch (carbohydrate) that resists digestion in the small intestine.

- ⊙ **RESTLESS LEGS** – A medical condition where there is an urge to move the legs. Described by individuals as pain, numbness, cramps, and many times as an indescribable sensation. Improves with walking.

- ➔ **RUTABAGAS** – A root vegetable similar to a turnip.
- ➔ **SADZA** – A cooked corn-based food that is staple food in Zimbabwe.
- ➔ **SECALINS** – A glycoprotein found in rye grain having gluten-like properties.
- ➔ **SLEEP APNEA** – Medical condition where there is lack of air flow to the lungs due to the lack of respiratory effort or airway obstruction of the nose, pharynx, or the base of the tongue. Can result in a lowering of oxygen throughout the night.
- ➔ **SORGHUM** – A grain of the grass family.
- ➔ **STEROIDAL LACTONE** – A group of naturally occurring steroids that may help with inflammation.
- ➔ **TEMPEH** – And Indonesian food made from fermented soybeans.
- ➔ **TURMERIC** – Made from curcumin rhizome, alternate name.
- ➔ **TRANS FATS** – A type of unsaturated fat, may occur naturally in milk and meats. It can be produced artificially which can be deleterious to the body.
- ➔ **VALERENIC ACID** – Extracted from the Valerian plant, can be used as an herbal sedative.
- ➔ **VILLOUS** – Having villi, minute projections from the mucous membrane of the small intestine. The projections increase absorption area.
- ➔ **WITHANOLIDES** – Natural steroid with a steroid backbone bone attached to lactone.

TIPS AND RECIPES

We need to establish a gradual change and progress slowly into a new way of eating. Even the individual food items will change. Some of you are already practicing healthy eating habits which is commendable. However, health advice is a dime a dozen. If the so-called experts get it wrong, then how are you going to navigate the sea of information when some advice is simply wrong?

You're about to embark on a journey to change your entire way of looking at food, exercise, and dealing with stress. The change cannot occur overnight. Some people are so motivated that they can make a "cold turkey" dramatic change, but let's be honest, most of us would not want the change to occur so rapidly. The DES concepts are a three-step process that should progress in a way that you can accommodate the changes at your own pace. You must give up certain foods immediately, which I believe is the hardest part.

REARRANGE THE PANTRY

Don't just move the prohibited foods to one side and promise yourself that you won't eat them again because I know you will if they are available!

Clear an area in the pantry and place all inflammatory foods in this spot. Then place all the ultra-processed foods in the same spot. The remaining items can probably be used in Step One or Two. Don't forget to clear the refrigerator and freezer as well. It is now time to go to the supermarket.

Remember Step One? Meat and vegetables for a week. No fruit, no carbs except what is contained in the vegetables.

SHOPPING LIST FOR STEP ONE

- ➔ L-glutamine supplement 1000 mg
- ➔ Probiotics: yogurt, kefir, kombucha, aged cheeses
- ➔ Grass fed beef for 3 to 5 meals
- ➔ Poultry, chicken, or turkey for 3 to 5 meals
- ➔ Eggs
- ➔ Your favorite fish for 2 to 3 meals, canned salmon, tuna, or sardines are options.
- ➔ Canned beans (soaked, pressure cooked beans, if lectin sensitive)
- ➔ Frozen veggies: peas, carrots, broccoli, cauliflower, okra
- ➔ Fresh vegetables, preferably in season, such as carrots, lettuce, spinach, squash, peppers (red, yellow, or green), slaw, cabbage, turnips, green beans, beets, and avocados (I know it's a fruit!).
- ➔ Unsalted or lightly salted nuts include almonds, walnuts, pecans, and pistachios
- ➔ Prebiotics: onions, garlic, asparagus, mushrooms, artichokes, jarred artichoke hearts
- ➔ Spices (none with MSG)
- ➔ Vinegar
- ➔ Olive oil
- ➔ Avocado oil
- ➔ Primal Kitchen brand mayonnaise
- ➔ Tomato sauce
- ➔ Salsa
- ➔ Cheese
- ➔ Butter (no margarine and preferably from grass-fed cows)
- ➔ Ghee, organic, homemade, or prepackaged in the oils isle of the Supermarket

  WEIGHT LOSS *with* DIET EXERCISE STRESS REDUCTION

BEVERAGES

Fruit juices are never to be consumed. You don't want to drink beer or wine during lunch. Water is just fine, but many people find drinking just water not very appealing. There are some alternatives. You can flavor the water with berries or vegetables, such as cucumber and/or lime. The fruit juices you have in your pantry, that you still haven't discarded, can be utilized by adding one or 2 ounces to flavor 8 ounces of clear water. You can also prepare green tea in bulk, say 20 ounces at a time and keep the carafe in the fridge. I drink my tea black or green unsweetened, but if you want yours sweet you can use monk fruit, Allulose, or Stevia. Nonalcoholic beer can be used, but only a few times a week. The barley in the beer has gluten and can cause inflammation. I really like V-8 juice as it is low in sugar, although it is high in salt. Flavored sparkling water is also an option, as are coffee, herbal teas, and milk.

SEED BREAD

Better Basic Culture TM is acceptable if you must have a bread alternative. By experience, it is best served untoasted at room temperature or warm.

PANTRY STAPLES FOR STEPS TWO AND THREE

- Canned beans
- Chicken broth
- Beef broth
- Almond butter (without added sugars) Almond meal flour

- Sweet potatoes (limit consumption)
- Coconut milk
- Canned fish: salmon, tuna, sardines, anchovies
- Canned peas

- ➔ Soy sauce
  or coconut aminos
- ➔ Rice (converted
  or basmati only)
- ➔ Quinoa
- ➔ Tahini

- ➔ Pine nuts
- ➔ Olives
- ➔ Onions
- ➔ Garlic

SAMPLE RECIPES FOR STEP ONE

Meat and vegetables seem to be simple enough especially for the meat, but what about the vegetables? You can only have so much lettuce with oil and vinegar. We have included a section on salads using various ingredients that should add some variety to your choices. If you remove the meat from the salad, you now have a nice brunch or dinner **meatless** dish. Remember that Step Three will help protect against heart disease and requires a reduction in the amount of white and red meat you are consuming.

SALADS

PREPACKAGED

These are particularly helpful on busy weeknights. They are sold with a variety of greens. Stick to organic, if possible. Some with a prepackaged dressing. Toss out the prepackaged dressing and prepare your own. Combined with your choice of protein, fresh vegetables and legumes or pantry items such as artichoke hearts, roasted red peppers, beets, etc. Ground flax seeds are a good protein source.

 WEIGHT LOSS *with* DIET EXERCISE STRESS REDUCTION

SPINACH SALAD

2 TO 3 SERVINGS.

- 1/4 small red onion, diced
- 1/4 cup sliced almonds, toasted
- 1/4 cup white or brown balsamic
- 3 to 4 strawberries, sliced
- 1 teaspoon salt
- 1/2 teaspoon pepper
- 1/4 to 1/2 teaspoon Stevia/monk fruit blend
- 1/4 cup avocado oil
- 5-ounce bag of organic baby spinach
- 1/4 Bosc pear, firm, thinly sliced

Preheat a toaster oven to 350°F. Place the almonds in a single layer on a foil lined baking sheet. Toast them for approximately 3 to 5 minutes. Monitor them closely to avoid burning them. Once they are lightly browned, remove them from the oven and set aside. Prepare the dressing in a serving bowl by mixing the red onion, balsamic vinegar, and salt. Gradually drizzle in avocado oil. Add the spinach, pears, and strawberries to the bowl and toss thoroughly. Sprinkle in the toasted almonds and serve.

ARUGULA, BEET AND GOAT CHEESE SALAD

2-3 SERVINGS

- 5-ounce bag of organic arugula
- 1 Beet roasted, peeled, and chopped
- 1/4 cup of roasted pecans
- 1-ounce goat cheese
- Balsamic vinegar dressing to taste
- 1/2 ground teaspoon flax seed for added texture (optional)

Preheat a toaster oven to 350 degrees. Wrap beet in foil to make a pouch. Roast the beet for approximately 45 minutes or until tender. Roasting is preferred as it retains the nutrients and makes for easier peeling. Once it is cooked, cut into 1-inch pieces. Add the dressing and arrange the beets, followed by arugula, flax seed, and pecans. Toss well. Add in the goat cheese and toss lightly. Adjust seasonings as needed.

Roasting is preferred as it retains the nutrients as opposed to boiling. It is a good idea to roast two to three beets at a time to eat throughout the week. They are available in orange and yellow.

AVOCADO CAESAR SALAD

2-3 SERVINGS

- 1 bag or head of romaine lettuce
- 1 Avocado, diced medium, lightly salted
- 1/4 cup sliced almonds or pepitas, toasted

DRESSING INGREDIENTS:

- ➔ 1 Anchovy filet* (optional).
- ➔ 1 large garlic clove, crushed
- ➔ 3/4 teaspoons salt
- ➔ 1 tablespoon Dijon mustard
- ➔ 1/4 cup of olive oil
- ➔ 2 tablespoons fresh lemon juice
- ➔ Approximately 4-5 drops of Worcestershire sauce

Place almonds or unsalted pepitas in a preheated 350°F oven. Toast for approximately 3 to 5 minutes. Monitor them closely to avoid burning them. Next, cut the romaine into 1-inch pieces and set aside. Add dressing to a serving bowl. Top with the almonds.

*Anchovy imparts a nutty flavor once combined

PREPARING THE DRESSING:

Add anchovy, garlic, salt, lemon juice, Worcestershire sauce, and Dijon mustard to the serving bowl. Mix with a fork until the anchovy has dissolved into the mixture. Slowly drizzle in olive oil. Add lettuce to the bowl and toss. Gloved hands work great to evenly distribute dressing. Add avocado and toss again lightly. Adjust seasoning accordingly. Sprinkle almonds or pepitas over the salad.

CRUCIFEROUS MEDITERRANEAN SALAD

2-3 SERVINGS

- 1/2 head cauliflower, roughly chopped
- 1 Roma tomato, deseeded, diced
- 1 7-ounce jar of marinated artichokes, drained
- 1 cup cucumber, diced
- 2 tablespoons extra virgin olive oil
- 1/4 cup lemon juice
- 1 clove of garlic
- Chili flakes
- Salt and pepper to taste
- Parsley, chopped (optional)

Add all ingredients to a mixing bowl, reserving the parsley. Toss thoroughly and place in the refrigerator for 1 to 2 hours. Toss and adjust seasonings as needed. Sprinkle with parsley before serving.

10-MINUTE MIXED LEAF SALAD

- 5-ounce package of mixed greens
- 1/4 onion, thinly sliced
- 1/4 cup toasted pine nuts
- 1 -14-ounce jar of artichoke hearts, drained and roughly chopped
- 1 red pepper, diced
- parmesan cheese (optional)

DRESSING INGREDIENTS

- 1/4 cup of grated parmesan cheese
- 3 tablespoons extra virgin olive oil
- 2 tablespoon red wine vinegar
- 1 teaspoon oregano
- 1/2 teaspoons salt
- 1/4 teaspoon garlic powder

Add all the dressing ingredients to a mixing bowl and whisk together until combined. Place salad ingredients in the serving bowl and toss. Add the dressing and toss once more.

CHOPPED ICEBERG SALAD WITH GINGER DRESSING

2 SERVINGS

- 1/2 head of iceberg lettuce
- 1 Roma tomato, firm, deseeded, and diced
- 1/2 stalk celery, paper thin slice

DRESSING INGREDIENTS

- 1 large carrot, roughly chopped
- 1/4 cup of rice vinegar
- 2 tablespoons avocado oil
- 1 tablespoon ginger, finely chopped

- ⊕ stevia to taste
- ⊕ 1 tablespoon white Shiro Miso*
- ⊕ 1/2 tablespoon toasted sesame oil
- ⊕ Salt and pepper to taste

Place all ingredients in the food processor. The leftover dressing will save refrigerated for five days.

*Fermented soy paste can be found in the refrigerated natural or health food section.

SIMPLE VINAIGRETTE

- ⊕ 1 part vinegar (may also be balsamic, rice, apple cider, red wine, white wine, etc.)
- ⊕ 2 parts Olive oil (may also be walnut, sesame, avocado, flaxseed, etc.)
- ⊕ Salt and pepper
- ⊕ A drop or two of Worcestershire sauce

Mix the ingredients in the amounts desired.

GREEN BEAN SALAD

4 SERVINGS

- ⊕ 1-pound green beans, trimmed, halved crosswise
- ⊕ 1/2 tsp. salt
- ⊕ 1 firm tomato, seeded, diced
- ⊕ 1/2 cup red onion

- → 3/4 cup feta cheese
- → 2 tbsp. lemon juice
- → 1/4 olive oil
- → 1/1/2 teaspoons Dijon mustard
- → 1 clove garlic, minced
- → 1 teaspoon salt
- → 1/2 teaspoon pepper

Place water in a large pot with salt. Once it is boiling, add the green beans and cook until fork tender. Quickly drain into an ice bath to stop the cooking process. Drain beans from the ice and pat dry. Add tomatoes, onions, and feta cheese. Whisk the remaining ingredients in a small bowl. Pour dressing over vegetables. Toss. Let marinate for 15-30 minutes.

CREAMY CUCUMBER SALAD

2-3 SERVINGS

- → 1 Cucumber sliced in half lengthwise, deseeded
- → 1/2 onion cut lengthwise, sliced
- → 1/3 of a cup of Greek yogurt or sour cream
- → 1/2 teaspoon onion powder
- → 1/2 teaspoon garlic powder
- → Salt and pepper to taste

Thoroughly toss all ingredients in a bowl. Refrigerate until chilled. Adjust seasonings to taste.

ZUCCHINI SUMMER SALAD

- ➔ 2 zucchini, sliced paper thin with a mandoline*
- ➔ ricotta or farmer's cheese
- ➔ Salt and pepper to taste
- ➔ Extra virgin olive oil, lemon juice, fresh herbs such as mint, dill, etc.

Lay zucchini slices on a flat serving plate. Crumble the cheese evenly over the zucchini Sprinkle with salt and pepper. Add the remaining ingredients to taste.

*A simplified handheld mandoline is a timesaver when it comes to slicing and shredding vegetables. They are available online for under $20.00.

BUTTERED CARROTS

4 SERVINGS

- ➔ 1 pound 1-2 bunches baby carrots, peeled and tops removed
- ➔ 1/2 teaspoon salt
- ➔ 3 tablespoons grass fed butter, salted
- ➔ Salt and pepper to taste

Place carrots with sufficient water to completely immerse them. Sprinkle in the 1/2 teaspoon of salt. Bring to a boil for five minutes or until slightly tender. Drain carrots. On medium heat, add the butter to the pan allowing the butter to melt. Toss in the carrots until cooked through and lightly browned. Season with salt and pepper.

ROASTED ASPARAGUS

3-4 SERVINGS

- ➔ 1 bunch of asparagus, bottoms trimmed
- ➔ 1 tablespoon extra virgin olive oil
- ➔ Salt and pepper
- ➔ 1/2 teaspoon balsamic vinegar (optional)

Preheat oven to 425°F. Place the asparagus on a foil lined pan. Toss with olive oil, balsamic vinegar salt, and pepper. Roast for 8 to 10 minutes. Remove from the oven. Adjust seasonings to taste.

CAULIFLOWER TABBOULEH

3 SERVINGS

- ➔ 1 pound cauliflower, grated or riced on a large box grater or in a food processor
- ➔ 1 teaspoon of salt, divided in two
- ➔ 1/2 cup of parsley
- ➔ 1 handful of mint
- ➔ 3 ounces extra virgin olive oil
- ➔ 1 clove of garlic, minced
- ➔ 3 tablespoons of lemon juice
- ➔ Zest of two lemons
- ➔ 3 scallions, thinly sliced

- ⊕ 1/2 cucumber, deseeded and diced in small pieces
- ⊕ 1 medium tomato, diced

Cook the riced cauliflower in a warm skillet with salt. Once tender, spread out and set aside. In the meantime, finely chop the parsley and mint or place them in a food processor, adding oil, lemon juice, and zest, and process all at once. Place riced cauliflower in a bowl and toss in all the ingredients. Adjust seasonings to taste.

CAULIFLOWER WITH TOASTED SPICES

4 SERVINGS

- ⊕ 1 head of cauliflower, steamed
- ⊕ 1/4 cup extra virgin olive oil
- ⊕ 1 teaspoon paprika
- ⊕ 1/2 teaspoon cumin
- ⊕ 1/4 teaspoon cinnamon
- ⊕ Two cloves of garlic, minced
- ⊕ 2 tablespoons fresh squeezed lemon juice
- ⊕ 1/4 cup flat leaf parsley, chopped
- ⊕ Salt and pepper to taste

Trim the stalk of cauliflower to the base leaving the pretty green leaves. Set in a pot in half an inch of water. Set to medium-low heat and simmer for approximately 10-12 minutes or until fork tender. Meanwhile, in a small sauté pan over medium low heat, lightly toast the paprika, cinnamon, and cumin until fragrant, approximately one minute. Remove from the heat and whisk in oil, add garlic, and cook a few seconds until garlic is cooked but not browned. Add lemon juice, salt, and pepper. Transfer the cauliflower to a platter and pour the spiced oil on top. Sprinkle with parsley.

GET TO KNOW NEW VEGETABLES. THEY ARE GOING TO BE THE BASIS OF YOUR DIET.

- Arugula
- Artichokes
- Asparagus
- Bamboo shoots
- Bean sprouts
- Bok Choi
- Broccoli
- Broccoli sprouts
- Brussel sprouts
- Cabbage
- Carrots
- Cauliflower
- Celery
- Chervil
- Cilantro
- Chives
- Cucumbers
- Daikon radishes
- Endive
- Eggplant
- Escarole
- Fennel
- Garlic
- Red, green, yellow peppers
- Collard greens
- Mustard greens
- Green beans
- Horseradish
- Jalapenos
- Jicama
- Kimchi
- Leaks
- Lettuce
- Mushrooms
- Onion
- Parsley
- Sauerkraut
- Sea vegetables

- ⊕ Scallions
- ⊕ Shallots
- ⊕ Spinach
- ⊕ Squash
- ⊕ Radicchio
- ⊕ Tomato
- ⊕ Turnip
- ⊕ Watercress
- ⊕ Yellow Squash
- ⊕ Zucchini

As far as meat is concerned you can consume fish, beef, chicken, turkey, and shrimp prepared in any way you choose. This is Step One that you will follow for one or two weeks, so the amount of meat is irrelevant. Do not be afraid of the fat, but keep in mind that this dietary change is temporary.

The following are some meat dishes that you may want to try.

GRILLED CHICKEN, SPINACH AND PORTOBELLO MUSHROOM SALAD

SERVES 4

- ⊕ 1 regular size package of baby Bella or button mushrooms, halved
- ⊕ 2 skinless chicken breasts teaspoon onion powder
- ⊕ 1 1/2 tbsp avocado oil
- ⊕ 1/4 cup toasted pine nuts (optional)
- ⊕ 3 tablespoon red wine vinegar
- ⊕ 1 teaspoon monk fruit/Stevia blend
- ⊕ 1/3 cup of olive oil
- ⊕ 2 teaspoons lemon juice

- ➔ 1/4 teaspoon lemon zest
- ➔ 1 teaspoon salt
- ➔ 6 cup spinach leaves
- ➔ 1 half thinly sliced red onion
- ➔ 3 tablespoons feta cheese

Heat a 12-inch skillet over medium heat and add avocado oil. When the oil is hot add the mushrooms. Allow them to brown one side then turn occasionally until they are uniformly browned. Remove from skillet and set aside. Rub chicken with avocado oil, onion powder, and lemon pepper. Allow to fry in grill or skillet for approximately 15 to 20 minutes or until juices run clear. Slice the chicken breasts diagonally. For the dressing, combine the red wine vinegar, sugar, olive oil, lemon juice, lemon zest, and salt in the serving bowl. Add the spinach and toss until it is coated. Place the chicken, mushrooms, onions, feta cheese, and optional pine nuts on top.

CHICKEN PARMESAN

SERVES 4

- ➔ 2 chicken breasts, butterflied or pounded to a half inch thickness
- ➔ 1/2 teaspoon onion powder
- ➔ 1/2 teaspoon garlic powder
- ➔ Salt and pepper to taste
- ➔ 1/2 cup Parmesan cheese or more as needed
- ➔ 1/4 cup avocado oil
- ➔ 1 firm tomato, deseeded, diced
- ➔ Small handful basil, roughly chopped

Butterfly or pound each breast to 1/2 thickness. Season with the next four ingredients. Be careful not to over-salt. Parmesan cheese also adds saltiness to the chicken. Press the parmesan on both sides of the breasts. Heat skillet and add avocado oil. Arrange chicken in the skillet without overcrowding. Fry in two batches if necessary. Brown on medium heat until juices run clear. Plate with the tomato basil garnish. A leafy green salad with basil, red onion, and tomato would make a good side dish. Season dressing with Italian flavorings such as oregano and garlic.

SHRIMP STUFFED AVOCADO BOATS

SERVES 1-2

- 7 ounces of shrimp, clean and deveined. You may also use cooked shrimp
- 1 tablespoon Old Bay seasoning
- 1 avocado
- Handful of mixed greens tossed in a light vinaigrette (see below)
- 2-3 tablespoons primal kitchen mayonnaise
- 1/2 stalk of celery, diced

Bring a saucepan of water to boil with Old Bay seasoning. Place the shrimp in boiling water. Cook until tender. Drain the saucepan. Cut the avocado lengthwise, saving the shell, score each half into cubes, and remove the avocado meat without cutting the skin. Chop the celery. Add mayonnaise to a bowl with the celery and cooled shrimp. Mix thoroughly. Add the avocado cubes. Adjust seasonings. Stuff the avocado shell. Place the avocado boats in a serving bowl or plate surrounded with the greens.

CHICKEN AND MUSHROOM STEW

SERVES 4

- ➔ 4 tablespoons extra virgin olive oil
- ➔ 2 garlic cloves, minced
- ➔ 2 pounds chicken thighs, bone in with fat and skin removed
- ➔ 16 ounces fresh mushroom caps, halved
- ➔ 1 28-ounce can tomatoes
- ➔ Salt and pepper
- ➔ 1 tablespoon of arrowroot mixed with 3 tablespoons of water

Add the two tablespoons of olive oil to a medium-hot skillet. Sauté until soft. Remove and set aside. Season the chicken generously with salt and pepper and add to the skillet. Brown each side well. While you are browning, add two tablespoons of olive oil to another skillet. Sauté the mushrooms caps on medium heat until they are golden, 6 to 7 minutes. Once the chicken is browned, add the tomatoes and mushrooms. Cook the chicken covered for 25 minutes, then uncovered for an additional 10 minutes. During the last two minutes, mix water into the arrowroot, breaking up any clumps. Stir evenly into the sauce.

Option: Add a bag of baby spinach during the last five minutes prior to adding the arrowroot.

MEDITERRANEAN LAMB CHOPS

SERVES 2

This dish is simple yet flavorful and elegant, perfect with a bright side salad made with balsamic or lemony vinaigrette.

- ➔ 4 Lamb chops
- ➔ 1 tablespoon lime juice
- ➔ Salt and pepper to taste
- ➔ 1 tsp oregano
- ➔ 1 tsp of olive oil

Place lamb chops in a bowl. Add the remaining five ingredients to the lamb and marinate for about 30 minutes. They can now be broiled, pan-fried, or grilled. For broiling, place 1 inch from the broiler at low for 4-5 minutes to sear. Continue cooking a few minutes more until your desired temperature.

SALAD SUGGESTION:

- ➔ Mixed greens or butter lettuce
- ➔ Raw asparagus tips (yes, asparagus may be eaten raw)
- ➔ Small mozzarella balls with vinaigrette recipe.

You may substitute lemon for vinegar.

SALISBURY STEAK

- 1 pound of ground sirloin (grass fed)
- 1/4 cup of almond flour
- 1/4 cup tomato sauce
- 1 tablespoon Worcestershire sauce
- Salt and pepper to taste (easy on the salt or simply omit)
- 1/4 teaspoon cayenne pepper, optional
- 2 teaspoons avocado oil, divided
- 1 teaspoon ghee
- 1 small onion, diced
- 1/2 teaspoon arrowroot starch
- 3/4 cup beef broth

Season the beef with the next six ingredients. Adjust seasonings to taste. Shape into small oval patties. Fry with half the avocado oil and ghee until cooked through. Heat the remaining avocado oil. Add the mushrooms and cook for 10 minutes over medium heat until golden. Add the diced onion. Sauté until translucent. In a small cup, mix arrowroot into a small amount of beef broth. Add the remaining beef broth to the pan and add the patties to reheat. Add reserved arrowroot and broth mixture to slightly thicken the sauce. Remove from heat. Makes 2 to 3 servings. Also, note that the patties can also be baked in the oven at 375°F for approximately 20 minutes.

SALISBURY STEAK NO-MEAT FOR STEP THREE

Use Impossible Meat TM instead of ground beef. Substitute mild or medium salsa instead of tomato sauce; use two tablespoons per serving, and you can omit the cayenne pepper. Add diced onions to the Impossible meat as well as the other ingredients. The mixture will be somewhat mushy, but if you spoon it and shape it on a piece of parchment paper, it will be easier to place in an oiled pan. Impossible meat cooks differently than real meat and requires lower temperatures. Low medium is usually hot enough. Avoid the ghee, and you can use prepackaged beef broth to make the gravy. You need to watch the salt content.

GRASS FED SIRLOIN

Grass-fed beef is leaner than grain finished ones. You'll have to adjust the way you cook the meat and prepare the meat accordingly. They will have to be treated differently. You can season it with onion and garlic powder, some olive oil and Worcestershire sauce. You can also use a prepared steak seasoning of choice. Let us take a look at some of the tips given by the experts. Marinades usually don't work with lean cuts of meat. You can, however, inject the beef so that the juices are added. You can also cook the meat first at a relatively low temperature (approximately 250 ° Fahrenheit) so that the internal temperature is around 120-125 °F using a meat thermometer. After you allow it to rest for several minutes, sear it at 500°F in a pellet grill, regular grill, or cast-iron skillet. This is known as reverse searing. It is also recommended that you let it sit for at least 10-15 minutes. If you let it sit any longer, it will become cold.

Seafood dishes can be consumed at all times during all three steps of the DES diet. Different preparation styles and different recipes tend to add variety to the palate. Here are some of our favorites.

    WEIGHT LOSS *with* DIET EXERCISE STRESS REDUCTION

HERB BAKED SALMON

3 SERVINGS

- 3/4 pounds of fresh wild salmon filet
- 2 cloves of garlic, sliced or crushed
- 1 teaspoon fresh rosemary, minced
- 1/2 teaspoon fresh or dried oregano
- 4 tablespoon ghee, melted
- 1 teaspoon lemon
- Salt and pepper to taste

Preheat oven to 400°F. Cut a large sheet of aluminum foil large enough to wrap the salmon. Spray the aluminum with coconut or avocado cooking spray. Pat the salmon dry. In a small bowl mix the salt, pepper, garlic, oregano, and ghee. Spread the mixture on the fish. Add the lemon juice on top. Wrap the fish entirely in the foil and place on a baking sheet. Cook for 15 minutes. Uncover and broil on top rack until the desired temperature is reached.

LEMON BUTTER SCALLOPS

- 1 pound large scallops
- 1 tablespoon olive oil
- 2 tablespoons butter, divided
- Salt and pepper
- 2 cloves of garlic, diced
- 1 tablespoon lemon juice
- Parsley for garnish

Dry scallops well. Add one tablespoon of butter and olive oil to a heated skillet. Once it is very hot; but not smoking, sprinkle salt and pepper on the scallops and sear on both sides. That usually takes 1 to 2 minutes on each side. Do not overcrowd the pan as they will not brown. A brown crust will form on both sides of the scallops. Remove scallops from the skillet. Reduce heat to medium and add the remaining butter and garlic. Cook until garlic is tender, then add lemon juice. Return the scallops to the sauce. Flip over several times to coat the scallops. Garnish with parsley

BAKED HALIBUT

SERVES 2

- 8 ounces of halibut
- Handful cherry tomatoes
- Two garlic cloves thinly slice on a mandolin or grated
- 1/4 teaspoon lemon zest
- Extra virgin olive oil
- Lemon juice, optional
- Salt and pepper to taste

Preheat oven to 35 0°F. Pat the halibut dry. Place it on a baking pan and sprinkle with lemon zest. Slice the cherry tomatoes in half. Toss together with the garlic. Add them to the baking pan surrounding the fish. Season the fish and tomatoes with salt and pepper to taste. Drizzle with olive oil and bake for approximately 10 to 12 minutes.

 WEIGHT LOSS *with* DIET EXERCISE STRESS REDUCTION

SOUTHWEST SOCKEYE SALMON

SERVES 4

- ➔ 16-ounce salmon filet
- ➔ Avocado oil

RUB:

- ➔ Chili powder
- ➔ Smoked paprika
- ➔ Garlic powder
- ➔ Cumin
- ➔ Pepper
- ➔ Celery salt or kosher salt

Rub the fish with a liberal amount of avocado oil. Season to taste with the remaining rub ingredients. The fish is easy to prepare and can be pan-fried or grilled. Just be sure to clean and oil your grill grates. The leftover rub can be used again for other dishes.

NO CARB NIÇOISES STYLE TUNA SALAD

SERVES 2

- ➔ 5-ounces combined lettuce (Boston, romaine, iceberg, butter) chopped into bite size pieces

- ⊙ 1 can of canned tuna

- ⊙ 1/4 red onion, diced

- ⊙ 2 tablespoons red wine vinegar mixed with 1 tablespoon of water

- ⊙ 1 teaspoon of kosher salt

- ⊙ 1 teaspoon of Dijon mustard

- ⊙ 1 teaspoon fresh ground pepper

- ⊙ 1/4 cup of olive oil

- ⊙ 1/4 cup combination of olives, such as cerignola, Niçoises, Kalamata, etc.

- ⊙ 1/4 cup small red pepper, diced

- ⊙ 1/2 cup butternut squash, roasted

- ⊙ 1/2 cup French green beans, cut into 1 inch pieces

- ⊙ 1 teaspoon of capers

- ⊙ 1 hardboiled egg, sliced

Prepare the dressing by placing the onion, vinegar, water, mustard, salt, and pepper in the serving bowl until the salt is dissolved and allowing the onion to marinate. Cook the green beans in salted water for approximately 10 minutes or until tender. Let cool. Slowly whisk in the olive oil into the vinegar mixture until it is emulsified. Add the chopped lettuce, olives, red peppers, green beans, squash, and capers to the bowl. Toss and adjust seasonings as necessary. Top with tuna and a hard-boiled egg.

MEATLESS DISHES

The meatless dishes will be the most difficult to get used to. Going carb-less is a little easier as the meat dishes with vegetables are more acceptable to the palate (Step One). That leaves only vegetables with carbohydrates

     WEIGHT LOSS *with* DIET EXERCISE STRESS REDUCTION

for Step Two and Three, which, in a sense, is what vegetarians do. Many of us cannot fathom going without meat; however, it is easier than you think. **Remember, you don't have to stop eating meat altogether; just reduce the portions and the meals containing meat**. The carbohydrates that we recommend are heavy in resistant starches. The transition can be made slowly from meal from to meal and substituting item for item at your own pace. Let me give an example. Being from the Caribbean, rice and beans are some of our food staples. So, I have adapted basmati rice and, even though I don't like it as much, converted rice. You have to remember that rice can become a resistant starch if, after cooking, it is allowed to cool. If you reheat it, it still retains its resistant starch properties. So, I usually cook 3/4 a cup of rice, which will allow me to have three quarter cup servings throughout the week. When I reheat it, I like a bit of crispy rice in the bottom. Turns out that an 8-inch pan with a tablespoon of olive oil or avocado oil allows me to reheat the precooked rice over medium to high heat. Add a small amount of avocado or olive oil and spread it evenly in the pan. Just cover the oil with approximately a half an inch of rice. I cover it, and in five or six minutes, it is reheated, and the bottom is crispy. You can adjust the temperature and times, so it cooks to your liking. If it is one of my no-meat meals, then as it is cooking, I place an egg on top of the rice, cover it, and wait till the egg is cooked to my liking. I consume this with beans. A can of beans usually has three servings. I like to season the beans, spicy but not necessarily spicy hot. Another meal can consist of adding water to the beans to make a bean soup. Add resistant starches to the soup including millet, quinoa, or lentils. A tablespoon or two is enough. These usually cook quite readily within 20-30 minutes. A **few** pieces of leftover meat or sausage can also be added; a small amount of flavor is acceptable. You can then add some peas and carrots to the soup. This is easy because it comes ready in the frozen section. You are now talking about a bean soup that is quite hearty; because of the resistant starch composition, you will not be hungry for hours, especially if you down it with V-8 juice.

I count eating fish as a meatless dish. And every once in a while, I will, in fact, have no meat and no fish. The usual substitution is an egg for the protein. Legumes are also a good substitute. I have included some meatless dishes with no red meat, white meat, or fish. A list of protein content of some selected foods is included in Appendix F.

AVOCADO TOAST

- → 1 slice Basic Culture Bread TM or gluten-free bread (Schar, Uris, Against the grain, etc.)
- → 1 quarter of an avocado, lightly smashed, and salted
- → 1 slice of tomato
- → 2 poached or soft-boiled eggs
- → 1/2 teaspoons salt
- → 1 teaspoon apple cider vinegar
- → Micro-greens (optional)
- → Lemon wedge

Heat a saucepan with enough water to submerge the eggs. Add salt and vinegar. Bring the water to a medium simmer; before the water begins to boil, crack each egg individually into a bowl, then slide the eggs into the water one at a time. Keep an eye on the eggs. It will take 2-4 minutes to cook, depending on your preference. Remove the eggs with a slotted spoon and place on a plate. While the eggs are cooking, place the bread in the toaster oven. Once the toast has slightly cooled, spread the toast with the avocado, followed by tomato slices, egg, and greens. Top with a touch of olive oil and a few drops of lemon.

     WEIGHT LOSS *with* DIET EXERCISE STRESS REDUCTION

MUNG BEAN STIR FRY WITH CABBAGE

- ➔ 2 cloves of garlic
- ➔ 1-pound green cabbage, approximately half a head cut 1/2 inch strips
- ➔ 1/4 teaspoon chili pepper spray
- ➔ 1 scallion
- ➔ 2 eggs
- ➔ 2 teaspoons cooking sherry
- ➔ Soy sauce, to taste
- ➔ 1bundle of mung bean vermicelli
- ➔ Salt to taste
- ➔ 1/4 teaspoon of Stevia
- ➔ 1/2 teaspoon sesame oil
- ➔ 1 tablespoon of avocado oil

Soak mung bean vermicelli in boiling water for approximately 10 minutes. In a separate bowl, beat the eggs with the sesame oil, salt, and one teaspoon of sherry wine. Heat half the avocado oil on high in a wok or rounded skillet. Add eggs, scramble, and remove while still slightly runny; this will take about 20 seconds. Set aside. Heat the remaining oil in the wok over medium-high heat. Add the chili, garlic, and scallion, and cook for 30 seconds, or until fragrant. Before the garlic starts to brown, add the cabbage and stir fry until wilted. Pull the vermicelli out of the water and add them to the cabbage. Then add the cooked egg and the remaining teaspoon of sherry wine. Add the Stevia, soy sauce, and pepper. Stir fry about a minute longer and serve.

Optional additions: chopped cilantro coconut aminos in place of soy sauce, a combination of soy sauce, fish sauce, ponzu sauce, sriracha, etc.

SHAKSHUKA

This Israeli breakfast can double as a quick weeknight or weekend brunch. There is room for creativity by adding or combining vegetables such as zucchini, butternut squash, artichokes, etc.

- ➔ 1 tablespoon olive oil
- ➔ 1 medium onion, diced
- ➔ 1/2 red bell pepper, diced
- ➔ 3 cloves of garlic, crushed or thinly sliced
- ➔ 2 teaspoons paprika
- ➔ 1/2 teaspoon cumin
- ➔ 1/2 teaspoon chili powder
- ➔ 1-28 can whole peeled tomatoes
- ➔ 4-5 large eggs
- ➔ Handful of cilantro, chopped
- ➔ Handful flat leaf parsley, chopped
- ➔ Salt and pepper to taste

In a medium-sized skillet, heat the extra virgin olive oil. Sauté the onions in oil until they are translucent. Add the red bell pepper, garlic, and spices. Sauté the mixture 1-2 minutes longer. Pour in the tomatoes with its juices. Break up the tomatoes into small pieces using a spatula. Season the sauce with salt and pepper. Simmer for 5 minutes. Using a large spoon, create wells in the sauce and crack the eggs into each well. Cover and cook the eggs until they are set to your liking. This is traditionally served with bread but can also be enjoyed with sliced avocado. If you use bread, use gluten-free or seed bread. You can also use an almond flour pita.

 WEIGHT LOSS *with* DIET EXERCISE STRESS REDUCTION

MUSHROOM TACOS

- 5 tablespoons olive oil
- 8-ounce package of baby portobello mushrooms, halved
- Salt and pepper to taste
- Oregano
- Almond flour or non-GMO corn tortillas

TACO BAR INGREDIENTS:

- Thinly sliced cabbage
- Shredded Mexican cheese
- Salsa
- Avocado, mashed
- Onions, small diced
- Lime

Prepare a taco bar with the above ingredients. Heat olive oil in a large skillet. Add the mushrooms making sure not to overcrowd the pan. Cook in batches if necessary. Remove from the skillet when they are browned (I like them slightly charred). This will take about 10 minutes. Season the mushrooms with salt, pepper, and the oregano. Heat the tortillas in a tortilla warmer or a stovetop skillet. Almond flour tortillas do better in a skillet. Fill the tortillas with mushrooms. With the remaining ingredients, add the other flavorings in the amounts of your liking.

SPAGHETTI BOLOGNESE

SERVES 4

- ➔ 3/4-pound spaghetti squash (may also use gluten free pasta)
- ➔ 1/2 cup extra virgin olive oil
- ➔ 1 large zucchini, chopped
- ➔ 1 celery stalk cut into chunks
- ➔ 1 large, peeled carrot cut into chunks
- ➔ 1 pound cremini or white mushrooms, quartered
- ➔ 4 cloves of garlic
- ➔ 1/2 cup of milk
- ➔ 3/4 cup of red wine
- ➔ 1-28 ounce can of Marzano tomatoes
- ➔ 1/4 cup basil leaves, torn
- ➔ 1/2 teaspoon red pepper flakes
- ➔ 3/4 cup of freshly grated Parmesan cheese
- ➔ Salt and pepper to taste

Preheat oven to 400°F.

Line a baking sheet with parchment paper. Scoop out and discard the seeds of the squash and sprinkle the inside with olive oil. Place the squash on the prepared baking sheet flesh side up for 20 minutes. Turn the squash flesh side down and cook for about another 20 minutes. While the squash is cooking, coat a Dutch oven or medium sized pot with one tablespoon of extra-virgin olive oil. Strands of the squash should easily be pulled off with a fork and set aside. You can discard the shell. Place the carrots, onions, and garlic in a food processor. Pulse the vegetables until they are finely chopped. Add the vegetables to the heated pot. Add salt and black pepper, sauté until they are soft, approximately 5 minutes. Reattach the food processor bowl and add the mushrooms and zucchini. Pulse until chopped, but with some texture remaining. Add them to the pot with the remaining vegetables, followed by the red wine and milk. Stir occasionally until the liquid is mostly evaporated. Add crushed tomatoes, olive oil, and 1/2 cup of parmesan cheese. Place the squash or gluten-free spaghetti into individual bowls. Pour the sauce over the squash and top with basil and remaining Parmesan cheese.

SPINACH FRITTATA

SERVES 2-3

- 3/4 teaspoon avocado oil
- 1 half small onion, diced
- 4 ounces of baby spinach
- 1/2 cup of half-and-half (you can substitute with whole fat kefir if lactose intolerant)
- 1/8 tablespoon salt
- 4 eggs
- 1/2 cup of full fat feta cheese (cow or sheep), divided

Preheat oven to 350°F.

Heat olive oil in an 8-inch skillet until hot, add onions and sauté until translucent. Add spinach and sauté with the onions. When it becomes wilted, remove it from the heat. In a bowl, mix the eggs, cream, and salt. Add half the cheese to the skillet with the spinach. Bake until just set, about 15 to 20 minutes. Top with the remaining cheese. Cut into triangles.

Leftovers can be reheated as a simple yet satisfying lunch or dinner. It can be topped with baby greens tossing them in a vinaigrette dressing or simply a good quality olive oil and vinegar.

SOUPS

Soups can be prepared without meat. The basis for most of these soups is fresh almond milk. Unfortunately, store-bought almond milk is too light and too sweet. You can prepare your own.

FRESH ALMOND MILK:

For 2 cups of almond milk, soak 1/2 cup of almonds overnight or 8 hours. Drain the water and add 2 cups of distilled or purified water to the almonds and place in a high-speed blender. Blend on high. Use a nut bag to strain or two fine mesh strainers layered atop each other. Add the blended almonds and squeeze through the nut bag until 2 cups are yielded. You may add additional water if necessary to make the 2 cups. The milk will stay fresh for 3 to 4 days.

Different vegetables can be used to make soup. These would include:

- Zucchini
- Butternut squash
- Asparagus
- Tomato
- Basil
- Carrot

To prepare two servings of the soup:

1. Start by dicing half an onion and sauté in ghee or olive oil until translucent.

2. Boil or roast the vegetables using half the sauté blend.

3. Add almond milk to the desired consistency.

Some vegetables are denser and require more liquid. Season with salt. Sage pairs well with butternut squash. Melting cheese and tomato, pair well with carrot, as does ginger. For tomato soup, I recommend using Red Gold Tomato TM brand flavored with basil, oregano, and garlic.

SPANISH GAZPACHO (A COLD SOUP)

There are numerous gazpacho soup recipes in Spain. They vary by region. This adaptation requires minimal hands-on time and is especially enjoyable on hot summer days. The typical vegetables are listed below. You can get as creative as you like by adding or substituting vegetables such as red peppers. The recipe is approximate and should be adjusted to your preferences. It is relatively low in calories. Enjoy as a snack or as part of a meal.

- 1 box of organic chicken broth, chilled (there are low salt brands)
- 2 tomatoes, seeded and medium diced
- 1 small cucumber, seeded and medium diced
- 1 handful of radishes (approximately 8), quartered
- 1 scallion, sliced
- 1 tablespoon extra-virgin olive oil
- 1 teaspoon sherry vinegar
- 1/2 teaspoon of Worcestershire sauce
- Tabasco

➔ Salt to taste

Chill the boxed chicken broth in the refrigerator for at least 4 hours or longer. Place chicken broth in a bowl, add all the ingredients adjusting the seasonings as you go to taste. The gazpacho will save three days in the refrigerator.

RED DAL

➔ 2 cups red lentils

➔ Cups hot water

➔ 1/2 cup coconut milk

➔ 1 teaspoon avocado oil

➔ 1teaspoon ghee

➔ 1/4 onion, diced

➔ 1 inch piece of ginger, peeled and grated

➔ 2 garlic cloves, crushed

➔ 1tsp turmeric powder

➔ 1/4 teaspoon cumin

➔ 1/2 teaspoon garam masala or curry powder

➔ Salt and pepper

Optional garnishes: diced tomatoes, deseeded, chopped cilantro, lightly salted yogurt

Rinse the red lentils and let drain. In a medium saucepan, heat the avocado oil, and add the onion, garlic, ginger, and turmeric. Cook until the onion is translucent. Add the lentils and water, bring to a boil, and let simmer for 15 minutes. Add coconut milk, garam masala, or curry powder. Let simmer for another 10 minutes until it is near a porridge consistency. Serve warm in bowls and optional garnishes.

 WEIGHT LOSS *with* DIET EXERCISE STRESS REDUCTION

SNACKS (ALL STEPS)

- ➔ 1 medium celery stick filled with almond butter
- ➔ 1 hardboiled egg
- ➔ Turkey slices wrapped in large lettuce leaf with Primal brand* mayo and mustard
- ➔ Cucumber slices
- ➔ Cherry tomatoes
- ➔ Radishes, halved and sprinkled with salt
- ➔ Pistachios, almonds or walnuts, small handful
- ➔ 1/2 avocado, sliced or diced
- ➔ 6 medium sized olives
- ➔ 1-ounce hard cheese
- ➔ Jicama, sliced into matchsticks

AFTER STEP ONE YOU CAN ADD:

- ➔ Raspberries, small handful
- ➔ Blueberries, small handful
- ➔ Cherries small handful

*no sugars or seed oils added

While not a snack, the following simple recipe serves as a dessert treat.

- ➔ 1 8-ounce carton whipping cream
- ➔ 2 cups mixed berries (blueberries strawberries, raspberries)
- ➔ 1/4 teaspoon vanilla
- ➔ Stevia to taste

Wash all the berries. Trim the tops of the strawberries and slice them in half. Place a few strawberry slices in a medium-sized mixing bowl. Sprinkle with ½ teaspoon stevia and lightly macerate. Add the remaining berries to the mixing bowl and set aside. Meanwhile, whip the cream until soft peaks form. Add stevia to taste. Whip 10-15 seconds longer. Serve berries in a bowl and add whipped cream to taste.

REFERENCE SHEETS DR. BERRÍOS DES CONCEPTS.

FOR A PRINTABLE COPY OF THE REFERENCE SHEETS GO TO: WWW. DESCONCEPTS.COM

DES CONCEPTS SUMMARY

STEP ONE:

This step helps with weight loss and diabetes.

DIET: Start with a modified paleo diet which consists of meat and vegetables of choice. Modification to the diet includes:

NO CARBS   NO FRUIT

YOU CAN HAVE THE FOLLOWING: NUTS, DAIRY, LEGUMES, COFFEE.

Continue this part of the diet for a week, or two if you are very motivated. There are no restrictions if you do not have diabetes or very high, difficult to control cholesterol. You can start the diet if you are on a statin (cholesterol lowering drug) and may want to temporarily increase the dose. Follow the diet for only one week if you are on a statin. *If continued indefinitely, you could develop cardiovascular disease due to elevated cholesterol and lipids.*

EXERCISE: During Step One begin to walk one mile thrice a week. Perform resistance exercises twice a week.

STRESS REDUCTION: During Step One perform the 3/3/3/3 breathing exercises for 2-3 minutes daily.

STEP TWO:

This step helps with weight maintenance and diabetes.

DIET: Reintroduce the carbohydrates and these will now be **good carbs:**

LOW GLYCEMIC INDEX   LOW GLYCEMIC LOAD
RESISTANT STARCHES   HIGH FIBER

You will forever eliminate sodas, fruit juices, seed oils, desserts, ultra-processed, and inflammatory foods. Go easy on potatoes and splurge on vegetables. Acceptable oils are avocado and olive oil. Examples of resistant starches and root vegetables are included. You need to select a grain of choice as the basis of the diet. Basmati rice and pasta are good choices as they have a low glycemic index, but you need to be careful of the glycemic load (not too much!). Beans are a must and eat colorful veggies. You will eat just twice a day, brunch at 11:30 and dinner from 6 – 7:00 PM. Snack in the evening if you need to. Acceptable snack foods are nuts, chocolate (1 ounce or less), avocado, and cheese (small portion: 1 or 2 ounces). You can snack on fruit, especially if it is a berry. You can follow step two indefinitely, but if you have problems with cholesterol you need to follow step three and begin to reduce the amount of animal meat you are consuming.

EXERCISE: During Step Two, walk two miles twice or thrice a week. Perform resistance exercises twice a week.

Begin a program that best fits your schedule. I recommend 10 minutes a day. Will weekend workouts and exercising do? In the European Journal of Preventive Cardiology researchers found the "Weekend Warriors" had similar reduced cardiovascular risk to regular active subjects and reduced when compared to inactive physical patterns. Exercise longer on weekends. Just put your mind and body to it.

STRESS REDUCTION: During Step Two perform the 4/4/4/4 breathing exercises for 5 minutes daily.

Me time helps. Taking a Sunday nap, going to service has relieving effects. Take nature walks with the children, they could use de-stressing as well. Meditation, Tai chi, and yoga are all options.

STEP THREE:

This step is a diet only change that helps with cholesterol control.

I call this the half-fish diet. You do not necessarily eat half a fish, but rather you eat fish half the time. Do not forget that canned fish, shrimp, lobster, crab, and other shellfish count. You can start this step when you are ready and have adjusted to your new pantry foods. Strive for 50% reduction. It is not as difficult as it sounds; you consume no meat or eat fish every other meal. If you have 2 meat meals in a row, then the next 2 should be meat free or fish. On meat days, portions should be reduced (4 - 6 ounces), make them lean cuts, grass fed, skinless, and trim the fat. If you must have breakfast, exercise in the morning, and then have breakfast. Make it the same number of calories as the exercise.

If you begin to feel bloated, gain weight, feel fatigued or moody follow Step One for 2 or 3 days with no carbs.

ROOT VEGETABLES:

Beets, carrots, turnips, daikon, Jerusalem artichoke, sweet potato, cassava, celery root, parsnips, taro root, potatoes.

ROOT VEGETABLES BY GLYCEMIC INDEX: LOW GLYCEMIC INDEX G.I. (LESS THAN 55)

Carrots 16, daikon 32, radish 32, Jerusalem artichoke 32, celery root 35, cassava (yucca) 46, parsnips 52, taro root 54. These root vegetables are allowed during Step Two and Three.

BORDERLINE HIGH G.I. (CONSUMED SPARINGLY)

Beets 64, sweet potato 70

HIGH G.I. (70 OR HIGHER, AVOID THESE)

Turnips 73, Russet potatoes 76, boiled white potatoes 82, mashed potatoes 85, instant mashed potatoes 88, boiled red potatoes 89.

     WEIGHT LOSS *with* DIET EXERCISE STRESS REDUCTION

RESISTANT STARCHES:

Yams, pasta, Pearl barley, millet, whole-grain bread, navy beans, oatmeal (steel cut), lentils, brown rice, green papaya, farrow, turnips, peas, corn tortillas, cashews, jicama, sorghum, persimmon, celery root, green bananas, and plantains, precooked and cooled rice, taro root, yucca, tapioca, oats, quinoa, rice pasta, mung beans.

PROBIOTIC FOODS. These are the good guys of the microbiome (gut bugs!), and it will keep it healthy. They include:

Kimchi, sauerkraut, yogurt, kefir, Kombucha, dark chocolate (70%), Japanese Natto, some aged cheeses such as Gouda, cheddar, feta, provolone.

PREBIOTIC FOODS. These foods provide nourishment to the microbiome and include:

Jicama, dandelion greens, garlic, chicory root, artichoke, onions, radishes, leeks, asparagus, okra, carrots, mushrooms.

HIGH-FIBER FOODS:

FRUIT: figs, raspberries, pears, apple with skin, blackberries, blueberries, mango, guava, prunes, orange, bananas, strawberries.

CEREALS: psyllium, flaxseed, oats, bran flakes, brown rice, basmati rice, quinoa

BEANS: lentils, chickpeas, practically all the rest.

VEGETABLES: artichoke, peas, broccoli, avocado, acorn squash, edamame, collard greens, butter squash, cassava, olives, carrots, green bananas, and green plantain.

NUTS: Chia, pistachios, almonds, walnuts, pecans.

OTHER: popcorn, dark chocolate

AVOID AVOID AVOID AVOID AVOID AVOID AVOID AVOID AVOID AVOID AVOID:

PRO-INFLAMMATORY FOODS: THESE NEED TO BE AVOIDED.

Breads, rolls, baked goods, candy, cake, cookies, cereals (except old-fashioned oatmeal) cornstarch, cornbread, corn syrup, corn cakes, crackers, croissants, donuts, eggrolls, fast food, French fries, juice, snack foods, fried foods, flour, granola, honey, hotdogs, ice cream, margarine, molasses, muffins, noodles, pancakes, pastry, pizza, potatoes, potato chips, pudding, relishes, shortening, soda, sugar.

ULTRA-PROCESSED FOODS: 4 OR MORE SERVINGS A DAY IS ASSOCIATED WITH DECREASED LIFE EXPECTANCY AND SHOULD BE AVOIDED.

Custard, pudding, ice cream, ham, processed meat, chorizo, salami, mortadella, sausage, hamburger, morcilla, pate, foie-gras, meatballs, potato chips, breakfast cereals, pizza, margarine, pre-prepared pies, cookies, muffins, donuts, croissants, marzipan, carbonated drinks, artificially sweetened drinks, fruit drinks, distilled spirits (e.g., rum, gin, whiskey).

SEED OILS: SHOULD BE AVOIDED AS THEY CAUSE INFLAMMATION.

Flaxseed oil, canola oil, walnut oil, sesame seed oil, safflower oil, sunflower oil, peanut oil, grape seed, coconut oil, palm fruit oil, corn oil, soybean oil, cottonseed oil.